BELABORED

BELABORED

A Vindication of the Rights of Pregnant Women

LYZ LENZ

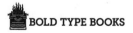 BOLD TYPE BOOKS

New York

A portion of "Context" originally appeared in *The Rumpus* ("Writing My Context," 2016) and appears here courtesy of The Rumpus.

A portion of "Miscarriage" originally appeared in *Jezebel* ("Why Are We So Paranoid about What Pregnant Women See?," 2016) and appears here courtesy of Jezebel.

Bold Type Books
116 East 16th Street, 8th Floor New York, NY 10003
www.boldtypebooks.org
@BoldTypeBooks

Printed in the United States of America

First Edition: August 2020

Published by Bold Type Books, an imprint of Perseus Books, LLC, a subsidiary of Hachette Book Group, Inc. Bold Type Books is a co-publishing venture of the Type Media Center and Perseus Books.

The Hachette Speakers Bureau provides a wide range of authors for speaking events. To find out more, go to www.hachettespeakersbureau.com or call (866) 376-6591.

The publisher is not responsible for websites (or their content) that are not owned by the publisher.

Print book interior design by Amy Quinn

Library of Congress Control Number: 2020001916

ISBNs: 978-1-5417-6283-1 (hardcover); 978-1-5417-6282-4 (ebook)

LSC-C

*To my children, who ripped up my vulva
on their way into the world.*

CONTENTS

INTRODUCTION

Who Gets to Be a Mother?

In a poem attributed to Herbert Farnham, a mother is described as a flower, majestic as a tree, gentle as the dew, calm as the quiet sea. She is as graceful as a bird and as beautiful as twilight. God, Farnham wrote, pulled all these elements together and called them simply "Mother."

I read Farnham's poem on a card that I received from my mother-in-law on my first Mother's Day in 2011. I was still sixty pounds over my pre-baby weight and constipated from the iron pills I had to take because I lost so much blood during labor. Every time I went to the bathroom, my bowel movement pressed against my stitches and made me cry. The only thing dewy about me was the noxious stew of postpartum juices in my underwear. My vagina looked like raw ground beef.

I tossed that card and all its treacle in the trash. What did those words mean, anyway? *Dew, sea, brook, flight.* None of them had any relation to my life as a mother. The fragrance of the flower had nothing to do with the deep darkness into which I stumbled every three hours each night to stuff my bleeding nipple into a screaming baby. With the way my boobs, once A cups and now

E cups, hung like balloons full of sand from my body. The rippling brook sounded nothing like the *womp womp womp* of the breast pump, which in my exhaustion-induced hallucinations I thought was saying, "Bob Hope, Bob Hope, Bob Hope," over and over. The majesty of the tree spoke to no part of my hormonal acne or the way I'd stare out the front door and imagine myself running away.

"How does it feel to be a mom?" my own mother had asked me.

"Like myself, but fatter and more tired and with weird shit coming out of my vagina," I said.

My mom has eight children. By the time she was the age I was when my daughter was born, she was already five kids deep. I don't think she'd forgotten what it felt like to be in my position. But she had done it all alone. Her own mother absent. My father working all the time. The burning pain of mastitis, the exhaustion, the times she must have sobbed in the bathroom because we wouldn't stop crying—it all had to be for something more than our fat upper pubic area.

A video from 2014 that went viral shows clips of job interviews for a position called Director of Operations. The applicants are told the job involves long hours, no pay, no sitting, no breaks and requires expertise in the culinary arts, medicine, and finance. The job, they are told at the end of the interview, is Mom.

The video, titled #WorldsToughestJob, has been viewed over twenty-eight million times. It is meant to be a celebration of motherhood. Of the pain and the struggle. A glorification of the brutalization of our bodies and the lack of help we get from our own partners and government. It says to women that this, *this* is the greatest thing you can be: a martyr, a mother.

The pedestal on top of which sits the perfect mother appears in our creation myths. There is Gaia, Mother Earth from Greek mythology, who bore the powerful monstrous children of the god

Uranus, the Titans. An Algonquian legend tells of the Mother of Life, who feeds plants, animals, and humans at her bosom. The Inca mythology includes Mama Pacha, fertility goddess of planting and harvesting. Christians have Eve, who failed in her first task—not to eat—and was given a second: bear children. Each creation story ties together the concepts of the worldly and the otherworldly. The flesh and the myth.

Not all creation stories begin with a mother. Not all of them involve a woman's body given up for the good of—as it's often phrased—mankind. But in America, to be a mother is to become a myth. To be a mother is to step into a role of someone else's invention, to cosplay a character who exists at the intersection of race, class, gender, and religion. Stepping into this role, a woman is no longer a human. (But then, was she ever truly seen as human?) She is now a river, she is dew, she is a majestic tree, she is earth and wind and magic and mama.

But not all mothers are permitted to embody this hallowed, all-consuming role. And who our culture sees as not succeeding in the role of mother says even more about how we conceive of mothers, than who we laud as perfect exemplars.

In our cultural imagination the perfect mother is a white, middle-class, straight, cisgender, married woman. She announces her pregnancy on social media with a photo in which she's smiling, draped in a gauzy dress, framing an almost nonexistent bump with her hands, wedding band glinting in the light. We are happy for her. We say, "Congrats," over and over in the comments. Her hair is perfectly curled. Her husband smiles benignly behind her. She is the modern-day Virgin Mary.

This mother doesn't force us to think of the complications of sperm and egg. With the focus on her glowing skin and hair, we get to skip that part. The perfect mother would never force us to think about sex.

Imagine if that woman had conceived before she was married, perhaps as a teenager. She announces she's pregnant and we whisper: "What happened? Couldn't she keep her legs closed? What went wrong?" We think of the darkness. We picture the wet-stained sheets. The tearful acceptance. Her parents. We blame her—her cavernous need. Her cavernous stupidity. We blame her, for her failure to live up to an arbitrary moral code. We don't reckon with the societal conditions. What we told (or didn't tell) her about conception. (After all, Texas, with its focus on abstinence-only education, has one of the highest teen pregnancy rates in the nation.[1]) We excuse the boy who refused to wear a condom, but not the girl who didn't push back and insist he wear it. The girl who didn't have access to birth control or who was too ashamed to seek it because of her religion, her family, her lack of money or adequate sex ed or both. No, in those moments we think only of the girl, of her sex.

Imagine she's black. (Why did we imagine her white in the first place?) Then our whispers silence and in their place are wry smiles. "Of course," we nod. "Of course *she's* pregnant." And, no, no, no, no, that nod doesn't make us racist. It's just statistics. It's not racist if it's a fact, right?

Imagine she has no husband. Imagine her husband is her wife. Imagine she has no uterus. Imagine her husband has a uterus and is carrying their child.

Imagine mothers.

America scorns a fat mother. In 2019, writer Virginia Sole-Smith reported in a story for *New York Times Magazine* that fertility clinics will refuse to work with women if they deem their body mass index (BMI) is too high. The science behind that reasoning is based on a 1952 study that associated obesity with "menstrual disturbances," a broad descriptor. Recent studies seem to back up the finding that women with higher weights have a harder time conceiving. But being "overweight" alone does not preclude conception or childbirth, and weight loss doesn't always guarantee success.[2]

In 2018, Dr. Mark Turrentine, chair of the committee that produced the American College of Obstetricians and Gynecologists' guidance on obesity and pregnancy, told the *Huffington Post* that the statistics surrounding pregnancy and weight need context to be fully understood. Although increased weight can be a complicating factor, the majority of overweight women have very healthy pregnancies. "Some of those potential risks, although they're increased compared to normal-weight women, they're still at a lower percentage," Turrentine said. "We're not saying there's this great high rate of complications."[3]

Roughly, over half of pregnant women in America are classified as obese.[4] When a woman the medical establishment determines is obese becomes pregnant, the risk we should be concerned about is not the risk to the fetus but the risk that the mother won't be treated as fully human. Study after study shows that doctors routinely discriminate against overweight women. A doctor's inability to see the woman for the weight means they often miss warning signs, which increases the risk of complications. What we should be asking is, What if it's not the woman and her weight that are the problem but the way she's seen by her doctors?

Our society refuses to see a fat person as anything other than someone who is selfish and depraved, lost to the sins of laziness and overeating. Media stories take a condescending, lecturing overtone. Mothers who are overweight are depicted as gross food addicts who risk their babies' lives with their refusal to lose weight. A fat mother who faces poor birth outcomes is held up as a cautionary tale for women who dare to be fat.

If a fat woman is allowed to become a mother, we certainly don't allow her to be a good mother. Her food choices and the food choices of her children are scrutinized, examined, silently judged. If she is a mother, she mustn't be a happy mother. She must always be trying to lose weight, always be struggling to model "healthy" behavior to her children, which is coded language for not eating, for not enjoying herself or her body.

America has a problem with fat mothers.

When Diane Delgado gave birth to her daughter in prison, she was shackled to the bed. Her legs and arms were immobilized. She couldn't move, even as the labor pains crashed over her. The metal cuffs cut into her skin, leaving her with bruises that lasted for three weeks. Even when she was given an epidural, no one loosened her restraints. She had to twist her body and hope she could hold still in that unnatural position while the anesthesiologist pushed the needle into her spine.

Even when the doctor asked the guards to remove her chains, they refused. "It's procedure and policy," she recalls them insisting. "Can't do it."[5]

In 2017, around 225,060 women in the United States were imprisoned in state and federal prisons and jails, and over a million more were on probation or parole.[6] In 2019, approximately 1,400 incarcerated women were pregnant.[7] Giving birth in prison is a horrific experience, both physically and emotionally. Prisoners have recounted being shackled to the bed, and many say they weren't allowed to have anyone in the room with them other than the hospital staff. One in eight incarcerated parents will lose their parental rights. And incarcerated mothers are the most likely to lose their children to foster care.[8]

The 1997 Adoption and Safe Families Act (ASFA) requires states to terminate parental rights for children who have been in foster care for fifteen of the last twenty-two months. According to the American Medical Association's *Journal of Ethics*, "Because the average sentence for women in prison is 18 months, by the time parents are released it is likely they will no longer have custody of their children. Thus, a sentence as short as 15 months can result in the lifelong separation of a mother and her children."[9]

Most of these women are not violent offenders. They are often in jail for petty theft or issues relating to mental health or addiction. As a by-product of the institutionalized racism, including generational wealth gaps, the black-coded "welfare queen" myth used to justify cutting social services, and the prejudiced policing and justice systems, these women are more likely to be women of color. Over 60 percent of women in state prisons have children younger than the age of eighteen.[10]

America does not allow women in jail to be mothers.

Shalon Irving was thirty-six when she had her first baby. Irving worked as an epidemiologist for the Centers for Disease Control and Prevention (CDC) and had a dual doctorate in sociology and gerontology. Her family described her as "an accomplished author and talented chef; skilled photographer and inveterate world traveler; and an ecstatic mother-to-be."[11]

Throughout her pregnancy, Irving, according to her mother Wanda, did everything right. When she found out she was pregnant while in Puerto Rico working to combat the Zika outbreak, she immediately got tested and confirmed she was negative for the virus. Over the course of her pregnancy, she was careful to take medication for a genetic condition she had that increased her risk of blood clots, and she never missed a doctor appointment. Irving had a detailed birth plan, down to who could be in the room, what conversations they could have, and what music could be played. That is the kind of woman Irving was: smart, detail-oriented, organized. And that was the kind of mother she would have been, had she been allowed to live. Irving gave birth to her baby, Soleil, in January 2017, via cesarean section. Everything was perfect, until Irving went home.

At home, Irving had trouble with her bladder, and though most mothers lose weight postpartum, Irving gained weight. She also had headaches and swollen legs. Again and again, she went back to the doctor, who—again and again—told her she was fine and this was normal. On January 21, only five hours after seeing her doctor and being told to "give it more time," Irving collapsed.[12] She was taken to the hospital, where, one week later, she was removed from life support. Despite having known risk factors that warranted a high level of care and attention, she died of preventable complications of high blood pressure.[13]

Maternal death is on the rise in the United States. The CDC estimates that 700 to 900 new and expectant mothers die in this nation each year, with an additional 500,000 women experiencing life-threatening postpartum complications. The risk of death is more than triple for black women compared to white women. Between 2011 and 2013, the mortality rate for black women was 43.5 in every 100,000 births compared to 12.7 per 100,000 births for non-Hispanic white women.[14]

Neel Shah, an obstetrician-gynecologist at Beth Israel Deaconess Medical Center in Boston and director of the Delivery Decisions Initiative at Ariadne Labs, notes, "The common thread is that when black women expressed concern about their symptoms, clinicians were more delayed and seemed to believe them less. . . . There is a very fine line between clinical intuition and unconscious bias."[15]

America is killing black mothers.

Black mothers who survive face discrimination and challenges to their maternal rights. America was founded on a system that required the surrender and oppression of black female bodies. In *The Negro Family in the United States*, historian and sociologist

E. Franklin Frazier details the systematic oppression and sexual assault of enslaved black mothers. Raped and assaulted, enslaved mothers were usually forced to abandon their own children to take care of the white children of their oppressors in the often-romanticized "Mammy" role. In *When Momma Speaks*, black theologian Stephanie Buckhanon Crowder explains, "Mammy epitomized the mind versus body, culture versus nature, dichotomy that would distinguish her from other African American enslaved women. While on the same continuum as more youthful, light-skinned childbearing slaves, mammy became the fulfillment of what a loyal oppressed woman should be: the blissful, asexual mother to children not her own."[16]

The experience of motherhood in America is a political question just as much as it's a question of flesh.

For decades, American doctors forcibly sterilized black, Hispanic, and Native American women and women who were poor or disabled to stop them from reproducing. Many women had no idea they were being sterilized.

"In the South," *Ms.* magazine reports, "it was such a widespread practice that it had a euphemism: a 'Mississippi appendectomy.'"[17]

In total, up through the 1960s, it's estimated that more than sixty thousand women were forcibly sterilized.[18] And America didn't stop regulating the right to be a mother with the surgical knife in that decade. In the 1970s and 1980s, doctors sterilized 25 to 30 percent of Native American women without their consent.[19] More recently, the Center for Investigative Reporting found that between 2006 and 2010, 148 women in California prisons were forced to undergo tubal ligations.[20]

As I wrote this chapter, Marshae Jones, a pregnant woman in Alabama, was shot in the stomach. Her fetus was killed. And though the woman who shot Jones walked free because she "acted out of self-defense," Jones faced charges of manslaughter for her fetus's death. She was being charged because she started it.[21] "It" is presumably the fight that preceded the shooting. But *it* is a loaded word in America. "It" could be rape. "It" could be domestic violence. "It" is what women deserve when we deem them deviant. The state of Alabama decided not to prosecute Jones after she was indicted for the crime by a grand jury.

In 2014, *The Root*, an online magazine, profiled three black women who had lost their children due to the simple act of trying to survive. The first, thirty-five-year-old homeless Air Force veteran Shanesha Taylor, was arrested and held in jail for ten days on two counts of felony child abuse because she left her children in the car during a job interview. She was able to reach a plea deal in her case, but others have gotten stuck in this catch-22.[22] Betty Brunson, was charged with child neglect after leaving her five children in the car while she retrieved a job application. Moshimalee Johnson, a mother of four, lost custody of her children after placing a Craigslist ad looking for housing.[23]

America does not allow black, or brown, or Native women to become mothers.

In a 2018 article for the magazine *Them*, Lara Americo, a trans woman, recounts the harrowing process of detransitioning so that she and her partner, a cis woman, could have a baby. The pain of being misgendered coupled with the societal misunderstanding and transphobia was crippling. She writes, "There is no version of 'What to Expect When You're Expecting' for transgender femmes trying to reinvigorate their penis."[24] Americo and her partner eventually conceived and had a child in 2019. Their story of motherhood is one rarely told, or considered.[25]

Transphobia, homophobia, and a lack of understanding about queer bodies' are rampant in our healthcare system. A 2018 article that examined a series of studies about the maternity experiences of lesbians who became mothers found that the women experienced heteronormativity or homophobia (or both) when seeking maternity care. This ranged from paper forms that assumed a heteronormative family structure, with a mother and a father; to difficulty accessing fertility specialists to help couples conceive without having a diagnosis of infertility (as evidenced by repeated failure to conceive through penis-in-vagina sex); to staff at the hospital barring the nonbirthing partner from the recovery room, even in instances when a male partner would be permitted; to refusal of care entirely.[26]

The Williams Institute at UCLA School of Law found that, in 2016, 114,000 same-sex couples in the United States had children. These couples, many of whom became parents through adoption or fostering, are challenging traditional ideas about what it means to be a parent, or a family, and because of that, they often face prejudice and discrimination.[27] Most recently, in 2018 Republican congressman Robert Aderholt added the Aderholt Amendment to the 2019 fiscal spending bill. The amendment would have allowed child welfare and adoption agencies to turn away families based on religion, sexual orientation, gender identity, and family structure. Although Congress stripped the amendment from the bill before it was passed, legal discrimination on the state level is still common. LGBTQ couples in America who wish to become parents face a complex legal system that often denies them their rights.

In 2019, the American Bar Association (ABA) attested: "State-sanctioned discrimination against LGBTQ individuals who wish to raise children has dramatically increased in recent years." As examples, the ABA highlighted ten states that give state-licensed welfare agencies the right to refuse to place children with LGBTQ couples. Many of these laws were passed after the United States Supreme Court legalized gay marriage in *Obergefell v. Hodges* in 2015.

America does not let queer people become parents.

The question of who gets to be a mother, and further, who is a good mother, cuts to the heart of our cultural biases and systemic inequalities. So, when we think of *mother*, we need to consider who we don't see represented.

Motherhood should be a choice—not compulsory, not restricted, but a choice allowed to everyone. However motherhood is chosen, it ought to be just that—chosen. For all the people stripped of the right to be mothers, more are forced into this role through abuse, rape, inadequate education or health care, and lack of access to birth control or abortion providers. So, when we talk about mothers, more than pregnancy photos and birth plans and which car seats to install in our minivans, we need to talk about choice. We need to talk about who is allowed in the delivery room and who is forced out. Who is killed in the delivery room. Who is forced in. We have to talk about the violence of the term *mother*. The way it cuts across and through our bodies. The story of motherhood is in so many ways the story of the female body. And what happens in and on this flesh is just as much massacre as it is miracle.

Throughout this book, I primarily use the terms *mother* and *motherhood* and female pronouns, in part because much of the culture surrounding pregnancy in America reflects and amplifies the misogyny our larger culture is steeped in. So, to talk about our cultural narratives of pregnancy is in many ways to talk about our cultural narratives of women. But I am also defaulting to this gendered lexicon because of the limitations of our culture and the English language. Although not all mothers give birth to their children and not all people who give birth to their children are mothers, *mother* and *motherhood* evoke the childbearing parent with a clarity, however illusory, that *parent* and *parenthood* do not, for instance. And because mothers continue to face higher standards and more judgment for their parenting than fathers do, *parent* alone doesn't capture the full weight of the cultural expectations placed on mothers. I try to use more inclusive and accurate alternatives where they exist, but I am sure I will fail in this. And my failures will feel constricting and limiting to mothers who don't identify with the words used. My failures are my own. And I hope that where I fail, others will succeed, showing us ways to better reflect the breadth and complexity of our reality.

This book is about pregnancy, but it is not a guide to your swollen boobs. This book is not a how-to for a gender reveal party. This book is an attempt to midrash the experience of motherhood. To plumb the depths and meaning of the text of our bodies. To look at the stories we have been told and to create new ones and better ones.

In her 1792 groundbreaking feminist treatise, Mary Wollstonecraft wrote, "I do not wish [women] to have power over men; but over themselves."[28] Like Wollstonecraft, I wish the same for all pregnant people. I wish for all people to be given the radical opportunity to have power over themselves. To have that power, we need to be able to choose freely whether to become pregnant or not. To bear—and to raise—a child is a radical choice that can reduce us to poverty, ruin our bodies, and compromise our employment, our earning potential, our lives, and our relationships. To become pregnant and to have children is to wade deeper into a world where your body is no longer yours, your body is debated by politicians, your body is manhandled by medical practitioners who won't listen, your body is a thing people in the Target checkout line and on the school playground and around a holiday table have opinions about.

To be pregnant, to be a mother, is to occupy a political space where your body is fought over and you feel powerless to control the conversation that rages around you. Power over our bodies begins with consent and consent begins with choice and choice is the primary right that is often stripped from people in their journeys to and through pregnancy.

Not long after I announced my second pregnancy, I was hired to be part of a team of mom bloggers paid by our local hospital system to blog about mothers and motherhood and pregnancy on its site. We earned fifty dollars a post, which, at the time, felt like a lot of money. The blog was called "The Real Moms of Eastern Iowa"—a send-up of the "Real Housewives" series. The hospital commissioned a glamorous photoshoot of us posing with our bumps and our babies. The pictures were published in a full-page ad in the hospital magazine and on mall kiosks, print mailers, even a billboard. We were beautiful, we were middle class, we were white, we were "The Real Moms of Eastern Iowa."

Less than a year into the project, one woman quit when she got divorced. I, too, quit, as my marriage grew more and more strained and the labor of the writing exceeded the pay. We were replaced by other smiling white ladies with children. It was like we'd never left, like we'd never been there at all. We were just placeholders for an ideal. The blog drew criticism from other mothers, who rightfully took issue with this vision of white, cisgender, heterosexual motherhood being cast as "real." The defense the hospital's marketing team offered was the same excuse you hear repeated in these situations: these are the mothers we found, they are the ones who'd write, we'd love to have diverse mothers, but they are hard to find. The reality was we were the women who could afford to take such low pay to write. We were the women who had the time to write.

Eventually, the project ended. The blog still exists but hasn't been updated since 2016; it remains on the Web as a clutter of broken images, broken links, and incomplete HTML tags. It's an online monument to a pervasive cultural ideal about what constitutes a real mother. An ideal that is shaped by class, patriarchy, and white supremacy.

To be a real mother is just to be a mother. And to be a mother is both a personal and political reckoning, a negotiation of culture and myth and science, an enterprise based more on survival than on who breastfeeds the best or the longest. But whatever else it is, it ought to be a choice.

Part I

FIRST TRIMESTER

Congratulations, you are pregnant.

Those two lines that appear on the plastic stick you peed on tell you with 99 percent accuracy that you are fucked.

Congratulations.

From this moment on, your body is no longer yours. Already you have Google-searched your symptoms and already you have typed "what should I do if I am pregnant?" Already you have ceded autonomy. It's not your fault; you've been trained to submit your body to the greater authority. Soon your obstetrician will weigh in. They'll give you a list of acceptable foods and medicines. Mothers will stroke your stomach. Strangers will comment.

You are used to being told how to carry yourself. How to dress yourself. How to be yourself. But this is different. Whatever little was yours is now gone. Lost to the life inside you.

Do it for the baby. Don't do that! You'll hurt the baby.

Maybe you wanted to create life. Instead, you will find yourself trapped in a black hole of expectations and demands. You cannot win. Abstain from all but the purest air and water and you will be labeled an uptight bitch. Say "Fuck it all" and drink a glass of wine, consume some caffeine, and you'll be told you're endangering your child. Everything endangers your child. High heels. Cold medicine. Working. Not working. Painting your nails. Not painting your nails. Eating too much. Not eating enough. Breathing. Living. Everything is a threat. You are the threat.

Politicians will decide when your fetus is viable. Politicians will tell you that you don't get a say in whether to bring this zygote from cell to human life. Healthcare decisions you thought were yours will be ripped from your hands. Vaginal delivery? C-section? You need to make a plan, but your plan rarely will be honored.

After, if you breastfeed, people will tell you to cover up when you nurse. Corporations will penalize you for taking time off. Childcare will be unaffordable. If you're a white woman with a white smile, ruffly blouse, impossibly clean white jeans, a sign that reads "Live, Laugh, Love" on your wall, and perfect blonde curls cascading down your back (*how does she do it, and with a baby?!*), strangers will smile at you and tell you you're blessed. But people will also tell you to use cloth diapers. Or disposable. Whichever one you are using is wrong. Whatever you do is wrong. You are exactly what society has told you to be, and yet, you are still wrong.

And if you don't look like that woman—if you are black, gay, trans, Asian, brown, Muslim, disabled, divorced, if you are a step-parent or you adopted, if you ever had an abortion, if you are on food stamps, if you are anything other than that blonde "Live, Laugh, Love" woman, whose name is probably Kynli,* your body has now become a war zone. It will be legislated, stared at,

---

* My apologies to Kynli, who didn't choose to be perfect but who was just born that way. Kynli, I am sure people criticize you, too, like we are doing now. See, you can't win. We can't win. Congratulations, we are mothers.

debated in public. People will ask you who the father is. People will ask you how you manage, how you cope. Maybe they'll tell you that you are a "hero," but it will be in the same voice that they say, "You have baby shit on your shirt." Or worse, they will say you aren't a real mother. You'll be excluded from the narrative.

Congratulations.

In bringing life into this world, no matter how you do this, you have forfeited your own life. Sacrificed your body on the altar of motherhood. Everything you do is scrutinized. Every mouthful you eat is watched. Every shoe or clothing choice is judged against the observer's notions of what is good for the baby.

Congratulations, you are now more myth than human. More of an idea than an individual. Now the most important thing about you is how you used your uterus. Now you will forever be defined by this relationship. Now people will send you cards with pastel pansies on them telling you *you* are a good mother. People will tell you that what you are doing is so good and noble. Then these same people will go vote away your healthcare, your paid maternity leave, your birth control—all while calling you #blessed.

"I don't know how you do it all," they will say, while also making it incredibly difficult to do it all.

Congratulations, and welcome to this magical journey.

Your body is a mystery. The landscape of your flesh is a region unknown to the very people insisting the loudest that they know what you should do. This means that your body is a palimpsest, written over and over by millennia of expectations and myth. The science of life is a dark art derived more from cultural expectations than objective data. As such, your body, now full of the kindling of life and power, ignites our cultural anxieties, over which we lay our desires, fear, envy.

Congratulations.

Conception

The first time I created life, I was drunk. My friend Anna had gotten married and I'd gone to the ceremony and reception, drinking wine and wearing a strapless silver dress with beadwork that slowly fell apart in tandem with the night. My then-husband was there, too. Sitting soberly at the table, regarding our carousing with suspicion. I don't actually remember it all. But I can piece together a scene based on memories from that night and other similar occasions. Me, loud, drinking and laughing. My husband, the staid one in the corner, eyeing us, disapproving. At that point in my marriage, only five years in, I still told myself and other people he wasn't disapproving. He was just an introvert. He was having fun, wasn't he? I'd ask him after every party.

Weren't you having fun? Weren't you?

He'd sigh. And say sure, there had been fun parts, but did I have to be so loud, or make that joke I knew he didn't like? Or perhaps he'd dodge the question entirely, instead telling me about something ridiculous he'd observed another person say or do. And then I'd sigh, relieved that at least I wasn't the object of his criticism.

He usually didn't like or want me when I was tipsy, with my blurred, sleepy gaiety. But it was the end of a long summer, during which we'd gone to Israel and El Salvador on vacations, and I'd graduated from my master's program. And now, here we were at this celebration, with my friends I'd known for almost ten years at that point.

And my dress really did look good. So did my shoulders, tanned from so much travel. And maybe he didn't quite disapprove of me all the way, like he would in later years. Maybe he still liked my laugh, still felt infected by the joy.

Of course, it could also have been perfunctory. Maybe I came onto him and he'd passively been like, sure, fine.

However it happened, it happened. Back at his mother's house, in the quiet of the basement room, where we were stashed away, chaos and darkness met water. Sex. I mean, sex. And we created a daughter.

He denies that this was the conception. He insists there was another moment. Some other night, back at our house after that wedding. But later, when I told Anna I was pregnant and told her my due date, she did the math and laughed. And told me it was from her wedding. A wedding gift. So, in my mind, that is the creation myth of my daughter.

Neither of those marriages lasted. Not Anna's and not mine. Perhaps that's why the creation myth shifted between my husband and me. Perhaps that's why in his mind it must have been another night. Something more reasonable and fitting with his personal mythology. And maybe that's why I am so insistent on it being Anna's wedding night. Because I believe I conceived our daughter in celebration. Conceived her on a night when I sat with other women—women who are still my friends and always will be, although the men are now all gone. I want to believe I conceived her on a night of friendship, lost silver beads, white dresses, and being wine drunk.

Whatever else, though, there was darkness and there was water. And upon that first moment of generative and formless existence we project a cultural narrative.

Before that moment, there were other times I thought I was pregnant. Once, early in my marriage, my period was late, so I went to Walgreens over my lunch break, came home, and peed on the test stick in my basement bathroom. In those anxious seconds before the test showed negative, I thought about what I would do. I didn't want a baby then; I wanted a life and a career. Still, I had a husband and a job. I was stable. I could raise a child, I thought. But I didn't want to. I wondered whether I could have a secret abortion. My husband would have left me if he ever found out. We disagreed over many things and abortion was one of them. He believed abortion was murder. I thought life was more complex, and that to imbue a mass of cells that may or may not have been expanding into life in my womb at that moment with the same weight as a child was overly simplistic.

The creation of life was something we disagreed about more generally. I believed the Bible was a myth. A powerful myth, but one that had space for science and the big bang. He believed in a literal six-day creation by a singular, Christian God.

If I had been pregnant, I don't know whether I would have known how to get an abortion. Or been able to muster the courage to seek one. To have one would have ended my marriage. Just as it would have if he'd known about the other time I thought I was pregnant.

That time, I was an undergraduate at a research conference presenting a paper on the hero's journey and my obsession with Joseph Campbell. I had been chosen by my professors for that spot, beating out two seniors. My school's English department was footing the bill. It was the first time my writing had stood out. The first time my writing meant something. At the conference, the night before the presentations, I was invited back to a room by some of the other students. At first there were many and finally just me and two men. We were drunk and got drunker. I am not sure exactly what happened. I know I made out with one. There are other flashes of memories too. My clothes are off and I want them on. My body hurts and I am afraid. I go back to my room and lock myself in. I remember the thick metal click of the lock. In the morning, someone tried to open the door. They shook the handle and pounded on the frame with a fist. They didn't mean anything by it, they yelled. It was just a thing. No one said my name. I don't think they ever knew it.

I lay in bed. Until they were gone. Then I looked up the nearest Planned Parenthood. I called a cab and overdrew my bank card paying for the ride. They gave me the morning after pill and I went back to the university, where I washed my face with Clean and Clear Morning Burst face wash. For years after, the bright, orangey smell would make me sick.

That afternoon, I gave my presentation to a full room. I talked about heroes and choices and destiny. I talked about how in Campbell's theory heroes can never really refuse the call. People clapped and told me I would be an academic and I bled into my underwear.

If I had had sex with them, then I was no longer a virgin. If I was no longer a virgin, the man I was dating would not want to marry me. But I needed him. I needed him in a way that a drowning person needs a life preserver. I had recently learned that one of my sisters had been abused for years by another family member. My family responded by doubling down in fear and silence. My whole life was falling apart. My family. My Christian upbringing. None of it was holding up to the harsh light of the truth. That whole year I was falling and falling and falling with the days. I held onto him and he was solid and good. But his goodness made him unforgiving. It required me to be virginal, holy, and pure.

If I had had sex. Even now, I can't bring myself to call it assault.

For so many years I pretended nothing happened just so I could live the life I'd later leave. A life that begins with a fundamental denial is, it turns out, no life at all.

After I gave my talk, I bled. I went into the bathroom and put my finger in the thick, oily blood, thankful for this darkness. This wetness. That was when I decided the moment hadn't happened. I would forget it. To survive, I wouldn't think about it. If I did think about it, everything would continue to break. And I couldn't handle that. So, I decided it didn't happen. I hadn't been expecting my period and didn't have a tampon. I shoved toilet paper up into my vagina, still so sore.

Occasionally, memories of that night surfaced in my mind. In the darkness. In bathrooms. In dorm rooms. When I thought about Joseph Campbell. When I thought about heroes. When my sister used Clean and Clear Morning Burst face wash in my bathroom when she visited. And in the basement bathroom, years later, in those moments when I thought I was pregnant. And the fear crept into me. That this small life in me would be the end of the life I had created for myself. The one I thought was good. The one where I was married to someone God-fearing, a taxpayer, a Republican, a Midwesterner. The one where I was a virgin, holy, good. The one where I cooked every night and bought throw pillows and spent hours thinking about paint colors for my walls. The one where I was the perfect mother. The one where I forgot the darkness and the blood.

The beginning of life happens in darkness. It happens with our eyes closed. It happens in pain, pleasure, water, and the formless shapes of our tangled bodies. In the beginning, the Bible tells us, the earth was dark and formless. The spirit of God hovered over the waters. Eventually, life would be called forth from this dark space, separated into binaries. Dark, light. Earth, sky. Land, water. But before that is a generative and formless space, about which nothing is known. Into that space we project a narrative.

To understand how life begins inside us is to reckon with how we understand life outside us. Eighty percent of Americans believe in God, and a majority of Americans believe that God had a hand in creation.[1] Whether we like it or not, the way we visualize the origins of life in the United States is heavily influenced by Christianity.

All over the world, early myths of creation begin with water and darkness. The creation myth of the North American Maidu people begins: "In the beginning there was no sun, no moon, no stars. All was dark, and everywhere there was only water. A raft came floating on the water. It came from the north, and it in were two persons—Turtle and the Father-of-the-Secret-Society."[2]

The Enûma Eliš, the Sumerian text that was influential in the creation of the biblical story, begins: "When there was no heaven, / no earth, no height, no depth, no name, / When Apsu was alone, / the sweet water, the first begetter; and Tiamat / the bitter water, and that / return to the womb."[3]

The story continues with the two waters, sweet and bitter, twisting and writhing together, in the convoluted chaos of prehistoric dark to create life.

In the Laws of Manu, a code of law that has influenced Hindu culture, life is created by the Self-existent, the "He" who, with a thought, creates water and plants a seed in it. That seed becomes a golden egg. The divine lives in the egg until he steps forth, breaking the egg into heaven and earth and spaces between.[4]

Science, which declares primacy, asserts that the universe exploded outward from primordial elements in a big bang of life. This swirling mystery began in a dark cosmos and eventually produced water, and then life. Darkness and water.

Of course, not every creation story begins in darkness. But from our origin stories come our ideas of conception. Though conception is not a mystery, the moment life begins is deeply unknowable from a scientific perspective. We know that a sperm cell enters a woman's body and fertilizes an egg. This egg grows and divides. Interphase, prophase, metaphase, anaphase, telophase, dividing and growing cells upon cells. But when do cells comprise humanity? How many cells does it take to make a baby?

The answer you give is more about faith than science.

A human organism is a human organism once sperm and egg make a zygote. But this fact tells us nothing of when a life becomes a human life, imbued with moral and personal rights and choices. After all, to possess life doesn't necessarily make something a human being, as we can see explored in stories of artificial creation, from *Frankenstein* to *A.I.* Science cannot tell you what makes something an autonomous being. All it can say is that life is present inside a woman. That a heartbeat is detectable at six weeks. Perhaps earlier.

Aristotle believed that the creation of a soul was a slow process—slower for girls than for boys—and only began at the quickening, that moment when the mother can first feel their child move. Augustine, the early Christian theologian who is credited with laying the foundation for Western Christianity, argued that a soul was created at the moment of conception.

Some rabbis have argued that the name of God, Yahweh, is not a name, but the sound of a breath. The breath of life, of God. This is when a child's life begins, when they take a breath.

As Randall Balmer documents in his book *Thy Kingdom Come*, conservative Christians used to believe life began at birth. The fetus, though alive, was not reckoned a soul.

What science offers are tools to track life. We have 3-D imaging, ultrasounds, fetal heart detectors, and more. We have data, but we don't know what it signifies. A fetal heartbeat is little more than electrical activity in a partially formed cardiovascular system. It's a collection of pulsing cells, necessary for the health of a baby, but not a full heartbeat the way we know it.

Still, politicians have projected a narrative onto this pulsing electrical current inside fetal cells to create bills that establish that personhood begins at six weeks—before many women even know they've missed their period.

At different points in our culture, the ways we have defined the moment personhood begins are as varied and as complex as our creation myths:

Life begins when there's a heartbeat.

Life begins at the quickening, when the mother first feels the baby move.

Life begins when the baby is first viable—and as technology advances, so does the point this metric defines as the beginning of life.

With the advent of new technology, premature babies that once could not have survived outside the womb can now live in small plastic chambers with IV fluids to keep them alive until they grow big enough to go home. Because of this, people who are pregnant don't speak of their tiny fetus; they speak of their baby. In an earlier time, they might not have known they were pregnant for months. Now, thanks to early pregnancy tests and ultrasounds, they can know they're pregnant within the first weeks after conception.

What was once considered a mass of cells lying in the darkness of a woman's body suddenly has a personality. It is a peanut. A tiny burrito. We attribute a disposition to that mass of cells with the electrical current. But this is a narrative founded in cultural mythology rather than in science, and it's complicating the language we use around abortion.

As I wrote this book, Alabama, Ohio, and Georgia all passed laws restricting access to abortion to six weeks on the basis of ultrasounds showing a "fetal heartbeat." I hope these laws are overturned, but I know there will be more and, in the meantime, people are being caught in the political push and pull. The language of these bills is calculated, designed to blend shame, religion, and science, a continuation of the Religious Right's 1970s tactics to shore up the moral majority in America. It's easy to get people to freak out about babies. Especially when there's so much about them we don't understand. The Right has intentionally created a single-issue voting bloc, one that allows it to control women's bodies. To control the means of life. Because the person who controls life controls the world.

In her book *Mass Hysteria: Medicine, Culture, and Mothers' Bodies*, Rebecca Kukla writes that the ultrasounds have publicized the interiority of a woman's body, that they look toward the fetus and away from the mother. Doctors and politicians, to assess a pregnancy, look inside, at the cells, and neglect to look outside, at the mother. Kukla notes: "At the level of policy, the insides of the pregnant woman's body are coming to have institutionalized public status quite distinct from that of the mother, and potentially in conflict with hers."[5] The science has been used to enhance our imagination of the fetus as a distinct being to the detriment of our understanding of the symbiotic relationship of pregnancy. And we project the fetus into the world irrespective of the person giving it life.

My parents took their eight children to anti-abortion rallies, and my mother made us hold signs, pictures of fully formed babies, infants that had clearly spent nine months in the womb and had been born. Other pictures, too, like the infamous one of the small, alien-like child in the womb, glowing with pale skin.

Other people carried signs with images of bloody body parts on them—pieces of babies who had been torn apart within the womb and then tossed into a trashcan. In all of these pictures the context was erased. The body that contained the fetus was just gone, a visual representation of a cultural divide that seeks to project a fetus into the world without the person carrying it, that strips the life from the means of life. In this way, the fleshy reality of the fetus is made more real, more viable, more human than the pregnant person.

It's not hard to imagine a future in which a mother's body is rendered completely unnecessary. Or worse, sacrificed for the baby through appeals to imaginary science. In Ohio, lawmakers are debating legislation that would force people with ectopic pregnancies to undergo a surgery to implant the fetus in the uterus. Except that isn't possible yet, or maybe ever. Lawmakers also want to force people with ectopic pregnancies to carry their fetuses until they miscarry. The medically advised protocol for ectopic pregnancies is to induce an abortion or perform emergency surgery because the fetus can't survive to term and the parent is at risk of dying.

In 2019, a writer for the conservative media outlet *The Federalist*, downplaying the risk of ectopic pregnancies (and ignoring the impossibility of viability of an ectopic fetus), asked, "Is that very small chance enough to prompt you to suffer through purposely destroying your own child?"[6]

The writer later apologized for her article after several doctors reached out to her to explain how ectopic pregnancies work. Her view is not how life works. But the same unscientific logic remains a constant, idiotic, and dangerous fault line that threatens lives.

To call a mass of cells a child and to pit it against the body that is growing it require an insidious logic that allows us to project a fetus bloodlessly into the public sphere. Ultrasound technology, while potentially lifesaving, has become an ideological cudgel in this fight. Stripped of their context and posted on billboards, ultrasound images become a kind of proof that is no proof at all. An unscientific foundation for pseudoscientific arguments.

A bumper sticker on a minivan in the parking lot of my children's school reads "Protect the rights of unborn women!" It's a trick. An in-love-with-itself inversion of a feminist commitment to protecting the rights of women. If you really loved women, the bumper sticker implies, you would love the unborn ones. As if it were that simple. As if assigning gender, personhood, and autonomy so soon was a matter of bumper-sticker-like clarity rather than an alchemical mix of mythology and cultural narratives. Of course, it's supposed to be clever, the shifting of the weight of a rhetoric onto the fetus rather than the woman—a cultural tug-of-war we wage, back and forth, in which all women lose.

This question of when a fetus becomes human reveals the messiness at the intersection of science, mythology, and pregnant bodies. There has never truly been a definitive answer, because the question is ultimately philosophical. No science, no religion, no myth has ever fully determined when a life becomes a person. In Justice Blackmun's 1973 *Roe v. Wade* decision in support of the right to abortion, he acknowledged this, declaring, "We need not resolve the difficult question of when life begins. When those trained in the respective disciplines of medicine, philosophy, and theology are unable to arrive at any consensus, the judiciary, at this point in the development of man's knowledge, is not in a position to speculate as to the answer."[7]

However unknowable the timing may be, the creation of new human life is a fleshy reality. I remember being afraid that whatever had happened that night at the conference would leave me pregnant. I remember thinking I would have an abortion, because it would have cost me too much to have had a baby then, at twenty. I also remember thinking I would never be able to tell anyone. So, I tried to separate myself from what happened. I tried to divide myself into parts. One acceptable, the other hidden. But the truth is that the story of our bodies is so tightly wrapped in the story of ourselves, we cannot separate them. The story of our bodies is also the story of our culture, our history, our science, our faith. They feed each other in an endless loop. To try to parse them out is to misunderstand what it means to be a human. More to the point, to pit mother against child is to misunderstand how our bodies function.

In a group of moms I belong to on Facebook, women shared their abortion stories. Situations ranged from rape and fear to complicated medical conditions and simply not being ready to be a mother. One way or another, these women had all found themselves there, regardless of whether they had used birth control.

On a larger scale, author Lindy West famously started the "shout your abortion" campaign for women all over the world to share their stories of abortion. None of them were simple. All the women who shared their stories of abortion believed that life began at different moments. Yet all were in agreement about their belief in the power of their own lives, their own self-conception.

If there was a theme, it was that conception and life, full human life, were two separate things, and that to conflate the two rendered the subject untenable. Pretending they were the same thing was an oversimplification in service of political ends.

For so much of history, women's primary cultural power lay in interiority—of body and mind. So, to dwell in mystery is to dwell in the power of women. This is not a power all women have, nor the only power women have. But in a system that devalues women, the womb's power could be crucial.

It can also be used against them. By separating that light and dark. That water and land. To create a binary is to strip pregnant people of their power. If the patriarchy can look at a pregnant person and decide when the fetus is considered a separate life, divide women's bodies into mother body and child body, they wrest power from them. It's a false dichotomy. But we routinely insist on dividing woman into parts. Legs. Ass. Thigh. Baby. All sold separately. It's incorrect—an error that disregards the biological fact that the body of the person carrying the child and the child itself cannot be truly separate. But sometimes facts are less important, and less powerful, than stories. After all, to divide the world into light and dark, baby and mother, is to exert control over the forces of creation. Let there be light. Let there be babies. Let us divide a body into two parts, pregnant person and child. Let us weigh the value of each so that woman and child are in opposition rather than in harmony. So that instead of symbiosis, there is discord. To divide is to conquer.

In 2012, Paul Ryan, who would three years later become the Republican Speaker of the House, introduced to the US House of Representatives a sanctity of human life bill that, if passed, would have legally established conception as the moment when life began.[8] Passing this bill would outlaw some forms of birth control, like Plan B, as well as all abortion. The bill has not been brought to the floor for a vote, but this isn't the first time such legislation has been proposed, nor will it be the last. Similar measures have been rejected in states across America, because they are still too unpopular politically and clearly unconstitutional. But this might not always be the case. The forward march of "heartbeat bills" and other legislation in various states means that societal norms and the constitutionality of such laws are constantly being reevaluated. And if conservatives continue to appoint Supreme Court justices, the line of what's unconstitutional in this realm could shift dramatically.

The righteous crusade of this legislation hides behind the language of science. Zygotes contain the potential for life, ergo they are life. So let us protect them. Let us tell women the who and the what and the why and the how of what is in her, whether we're right or wrong.

The body of a pregnant person must be a terrifying thing indeed if our entire culture spends every waking moment trying to control it, harness it, break it up for parts.

But life at its essence is resistant to binaries. Even after the umbilical cord is cut, is the separation total? After all, people who carry children in their womb give their cells to their child and the child gives cells to them—a chimeric system of interdependence. Who is in whom? I have two children and their cells live in me now and always. Even if something happens to my son or daughter, they will always be part of my body, in a way I don't fully understand. Even though they were born and are grown, I still have a hard time understanding where I end and they begin. I suppose they will too. And that's the tragedy and gift of pregnancy.

Virgin

On my sixteenth birthday, my father gave me a ring. It was Black Hills Gold. A yellow band with a heart made of flimsy pink and green gold leaves. This was my purity ring, the ring given to me to represent a pledge to safeguard my virginity. It was my commitment to abstinence. My commitment to God to keep myself pure until marriage.

Or, to put it more bluntly: The ring was a promise that I wouldn't put a dick in my vagina until that ring was replaced with a wedding ring. I hated it.

Plus, it only sort of worked.

Purity rings originated in the 1990s, right as I reached adolescence. Part of the True Love Waits campaign taken up by the Religious Right, purity rings symbolize a girl's commitment to abstinence before marriage. You were supposed to wear the ring on the finger where an engagement ring would go, a placeholder for marriage. You were to swap one constricting metal band given to you by your father for another constricting metal band from your husband. There were male equivalents, but they never caught on to the same extent. Nor did they have the same paternalistic element of being bestowed by a patriarch.

Purity rings are just one manifestation of a culture obsessed with female virginity. There are other manifestations, too, like purity balls and purity ceremonies. A creepy inversion of our cultural ceremonies celebrating romantic love that replace the husband with the father. As if one could and should be swapped out for the other. For a brief moment, purity rings were a cultural movement—Miley Cyrus had one, as did Jessica Simpson and Britney Spears. Under second President Bush, groups and organizations that promoted purity pledges and purity rings received federal grant money as part of the administration's abstinence-only education initiative.

As an eighties baby, my teen years were heavily influenced by the Christian counterculture of the nineties. Movements like True Love Waits advocated strict rules on sexual purity as a countermeasure to what people like my parents saw as an increasingly promiscuous society. They propelled Joshua Harris's 1997 book *I Kissed Dating Goodbye* onto the bestseller lists. Harris, a homeschooled kid, became the face of Christian counterculture by publishing a Christian magazine for teens and, at just twenty-one years of age, writing his book, which encouraged couples to save even kissing for their wedding day.

The book sold over 1.2 million copies and remains a fundamental text for Christians who want to encourage their children to keep it in their pants until marriage.[1] In 2018, after years and years of backlash and criticism, Harris released a documentary about the book with a pseudo-apology, noting that he never intended to hurt anyone, and ceased publication of the book. Then he got divorced and asked for privacy. I reached out to him multiple times for multiple stories I wanted to write, for so many outlets and also this book, and got no response from him until, finally, he told me he wanted me to respect his privacy. He built his career on telling others what to do, but, okay, now we had to leave him alone. His book, those lessons, have never left me alone. Even when I have begged them to. Even when I have not returned their emails. Even when I, too, have gotten divorced.

But at sixteen, I didn't know all of this was coming. I knew I didn't like any of it. But I wanted to be good, so desperately wanted to be perfect and holy and right. And for a woman, that means being pure, a virgin. So, I accepted the ring and wore it. I said "thank you" to my parents. And part of me was excited. It was jewelry. I hadn't received much more than earrings from Walmart at that point in my life, and I craved something that would give me the gravitas and glamour of adulthood. Anyway, what could I have said: "No, I don't want your ring—I kind of want to fuck around a little before marriage"?

There are, certainly, sixteen-year-olds with the guts to say something like that to their parents, but I wasn't one of them. No, I was a Type A people pleaser who just wanted to do the right thing, so much so that she'd wear a silly ring, cross her legs, and hope Jesus would save her purity.

Again, it only sort of worked.

In the Bible, the Virgin Mary is knocked up by the Holy Spirit. The baby is the son of God. The gospels depict Mary as a humble servant, willing and able to carry a child with no earthly father just for the glory of the Lord. Catholic tradition venerates Mary and has a doctrine declaring her perpetual virginity, as in she never had sex with a man, ever, despite being married to Joseph. Because of her purported purity, Mary, like Christ, is said to have triumphed over sin and been taken up to heaven by the power of the Lord. This is theologically different from dying, which involves a loss of the earthly and sinful body. In this theology,

Mary's body is sacrosanct and incorruptible and, thus, allowed to ascend to the heavens, whole and perfect. In a religion built on the idea that the stories of the Bible are not just true but also historically accurate, to erase the fleshy reality of penis, vagina, and some combination thereof reveals the patriarchal discomfort with female sexuality. The purity of Mary, especially prior to Jesus's birth, is essential in faith for the same reason purity is essential in American society—control over paternity. And she is the model girls are given at church: humble, meek, keeps her legs crossed, still has a baby. So we venerate her.

If Eve was the catalyst for the corruption of the female body, the vessel through which sin entered the world, Mary was the catalyst for its redemption, the vessel through which perfection entered the world. Both are bodies, both are conduits. One sinful. The other pure.

Most Protestant theology denies that Mary was a perpetual virgin, teaching that she had children with her husband after the birth of Jesus, which means she had to have done the old P&V—how else could it happen? Thomas Schreiner, a professor of New Testament interpretation and biblical theology at the Southern Baptist Theological Seminary, argues against the Catholic doctrine, noting, "Of course, Mary was a godly woman, but she was godly because God's grace rescued her from her sins based on Christ's atoning work. The only sinless human being was Jesus Christ. . . . By placing Mary on the same plane as Jesus, the matchless glory of Christ is diminished."[2]

Mary was good, Protestants argue, but not too good. She was holy, but not too holy. She was pure, but not so pure that it inconvenienced the male theologians contemplating her life. It's an impossible standard. This is the purity trap.

Where both Catholics and Protestants agree is that Mary's body was a sacrifice for the Lord—and that before her womb hosted the son of God, she was untainted by the touch of a man. After all, she could have never done her job if she had been touched by a man. What deity would want to come through the body of a slut?

Like with Mary, purity in American culture is more of a fetish than an actuality. We want women to be good, but not too good. Beautiful and alluring, but not slutty. To have sex, eventually, but not exude sexuality. Be pure, but still get pregnant. If navigating this line—really, more a moving target—is tricky for the mother of Christ, you can goddamn bet it's tricky for the rest of us. And it's supposed to be that way. It's supposed to be impossible. It's supposed to take all of our time and effort. It's supposed to keep us distracted.

In 1991 a pregnant Demi Moore was photographed nude for the cover of *Vanity Fair*. She's turned sideways, one arm covering her breasts and the other disappearing into the shadows below her belly and above her thigh. There was immediate public outrage. Stores hid the magazine's cover on the stands, as if it were porn. In an interview with film critic Roger Ebert from that same year, Moore noted, "I think more than anything else I was stunned at some of the negative responses. That people found it pornographic. . . . People think motherhood is wonderful, but it should be left behind closed doors."[3]

Here in 2020, though mothers are allowed to be more open about having bodies and desires and sexuality, if they do not hit that moving target of being pure, but not too pure, American society's condemnation is still swift and strident. Comments on Kim Kardashian's social media sites tell us all we need to know about how the status of perpetual virginity is imposed upon mothers. To one post from October 2018 that shows Kardashian posing in a vintage Chanel bikini, commenters responded: "You are a mom!" and "What do ur kids think of u" and "Lmao she's a mom." A look at Cardi B's Instagram story reveals more of the same attitude. In response to a post in October 2018, showing a clip of the pop star's music video "Money," commenters wrote, "I thought you were a mom #badparenting," "Stop selling sex and try covering up you stake naked damn you got a daughter," and, "love this Queen Mama like wow but stop this naked shit."

Of course, you don't have to look at the comments on celebrity mothers' social media sites to see these judgments. Stories abound with advice on how to dress modestly now that you are a mother; a multitude of Facebook groups feature mothers talking and sharing advice on how to cover up and conceal those parts deemed no longer appropriate to "flaunt." There is pushback to these ideas, but they remain a strong cultural refrain.

A relative once counseled me on the fact that because I was now a mother, I'd have to stop wearing tight jeans. Because what kind of model would I be for my children?

How did she think I became a mother in the first place?

At sixteen, with that purity ring on my finger, my virginity became tangible—a $29.99 circle of white gold. It wasn't the same for men. My brother tells me that although he was taught to abstain from sex, his sexuality was not a commodity for him to trade on. It didn't determine his value. Our parents didn't give him a symbol of purity to hold and wear and advertise.

Why would they? The ideal of purity is almost always associated with women. As Jessica Valenti writes in her book *The Purity Myth*, "Virgin sacrifices, popping cherries, white dresses, supposed vaginal tightness, you name it. Outside of the occasional reference to the male virgin in the form of a goofy movie about horny teenage boys, virginity is almost always about women."[4]

The female body, with all its caverns and spaces, is seen as particularly fallible. In the book *On Monsters and Marvels*, sixteenth-century surgeon Ambroise Paré chronicles the belief that snakes, lizards, and all manner of creatures could crawl their way into a woman's womb and impregnate her with a monster. He also recounts stories of women turning into men because women have "as much hidden within the body as men have exposed." He reasons, "Nature tends always toward what is most perfect and not, on the contrary, to perform in such a way that what is perfect should become imperfect."[5] Women can become men because, in Paré's logic, nature tends toward the perfect. But men would never be women, for the same reason. Women: imperfect, deceptive. Men: perfect physically and morally upright. As Paré unwittingly illustrates, men are afraid of the openings in a woman's body. Too many entrances and exits. Too many places they don't control.

The idea that a woman's virginity can be tracked and tested is one way to try to control women and their inconvenient interiors. But virginity is a social construct. It's not something tangible you can lose. There is no real way to test for it. Though there's a pervasive idea to this day that a virgin will have an "intact" hymen that is "broken" the first time she has intercourse, that's not the physical reality. A 2013 survey found that half of women don't bleed when losing their virginity. The hymen is, in fact, just a membrane that doesn't fully obstruct the opening of the vagina— how would someone who hasn't had penetrative sex menstruate if it did?—and it can be worn down or disrupted in many ways, from tampon use to horseback riding to running. Some are born with it, some are not. It's just a body part. Something like a baby tooth. How it comes out is sometimes a matter of force, sometimes a matter of gradual wear and tear over the course of living.[6] But what we tell ourselves about the hymen is perhaps more important than the physical reality of it. For women, it's the whole of our value. It's how men evaluate us, judge us. Entire traditions of marriage require proof of a woman's virginity through the blood of her hymen. That should tell you enough right there: we value a woman only through the blood she sheds.

Whereas the virginity myth that makes blood a badge of honor claims that once virginity is lost it can never be restored, the hymen can be reconstructed. The surgery is called "hymenoplasty." It's a controversial and medically unnecessary outpatient surgery. It takes half an hour and proves nothing except cultural bias. And even if a woman has a hymenoplasty, she might not bleed on first intercourse. A penis entering a vagina won't necessarily tear even an "intact" hymen. It's all a myth.

Of course, there is no virginity test for men. No blood ritual for them.

If virginity is not a particular physical state, what makes a virgin a virgin? We've yet to reach a consensus. If it has to do with intercourse, then what counts as intercourse? Oral sex? Fingering? Or must it be penetration by a penis? How far? And does it have to be consensual? Does all this mean a lesbian who's never been penetrated by a penis is a perpetual virgin no matter how much sex she's had? Do dildos count?

I remember these questions being debated quietly in the youth group at my church. Once, a visiting youth pastor spent the entire Wednesday night youth group session answering our anonymous questions. He passed around notecards, pens, and a basket. When we filled up the basket, he brought it to the front, reached in and pulled one out: "I had oral sex, am I still a virgin?"

The youth pastor had long blond hair and wore long shorts with a chain slung to the wallet in his pocket. He called us all dudes and slid his fingers through his hair before he spoke. "No, you aren't." Next question.

"Is it okay to touch myself?"

He slid his fingers through his hair. It was starting to seem like a nervous tic. "Dudes, stop messing with me!" he said.

But we were serious. I could feel it. This room of white, suburban teens wanted an answer. We wanted to know how the rules applied to our actual lives, messy and hormonal.

The pastor got angry as he pulled paper after paper out of the question box. Again, he accused us of trying to trick him. We really just wanted to know. Of course we did. We were trying to grapple with a question that had been debated from the ancient Greeks to Thomas Aquinas and up to the fight over abstinence-only education in schools. But we knew nothing of the history then, in that room—we were just confused, horny teens, who felt like we had invented our bodies; it was all so new.

Ancients, unaware of the biology of reproduction, naturally saw conception as miraculous. They organized into communities that centered around the mother.[7] In early Neolithic and Chalcolithic societies, the Mother Goddess was revered as the source of all life. Using the womb as the foundational force of the universe, ancient peoples created societies in which women had power and agency. The mystery of birth, hidden in the formless darkness of the caverns of a woman's body that waxed and waned like the seasons, offered an organizing principle that mirrored the patterns of nature. And it was often easier to trace blood kinship through the mother, because paternity could be unclear.

In their book, *The Dominant Sex*, Mathilde Vaerting and Mathias Vaerting argue that the ruling power creates the ruling deity in its own image. "The result is that the hegemony of male deities is usually associated with the dominance of men and the hegemony of female deities with the dominance of women."[8] Although many societies with dominant male deities also have female deities, the power between them is not equal. Once the myths reflecting a society's existing values are in place, they help sustain those values.

The early Roman traveler Diodorus Siculus observed that, in 49 BCE, women of Ethiopia practiced communal marriage and used weapons. In Libya, women formed the bulk of armies and served in governmental roles. Children were handed over to men, who raised them and nurtured them. Diodorus also noticed that in Egypt, where the Mother Goddess held her own against a bevy of male gods, women were accorded power, authority, and agency. "In fact," he wrote, "it was ordained that the queen should have greater power and honor than the king and that among private persons the wife should enjoy authority over the husband, husbands agreeing in their marriage contract that they will be obedient in all things to their wives."[9]

This matriarchal tradition was also practiced in Babylon, ancient Turkey, and Crete, where Spartan women, according to Nicholas of Damascus, "were entitled to be made pregnant with the handsomest man she could find."[10] Each of these societies found the locus of power and strength in a faith and mythology that venerated women.

It matters who your gods are. It matters even more who your goddesses are. In these ancient worlds, women ruled themselves and their societies.

Then came the pushes of war, the patterns of commerce, the spread of patriarchal religions, and these societies, sneeringly thought of as primitive, were erased from our historical memory. Although there are cultures in the world that are pure matriarchies, they are nowhere to be found in our cultural mythology.

Science is in on it, too. It's nice to think of science as objective truth, but it can be impossible to entirely disentangle scientific truth from the sexism, classism, homophobia, transphobia, and racism of the people practicing science in a specific historical and cultural context. Science can be used and misused to affirm or deny the experiences of women, people of color, LGBTQ people.

As with conception, we pretend we can define virginity scientifically, but these definitions are really driven by ideology, their true purpose being to divide a woman into parts. Just another tangle in this Gordian knot of our bodies.

Just like the myths are fiction but reveal the truth. Just like the birth and pregnancy stories we tell one another confidentially, over cups of coffee, on text message threads, and in parenting message groups, are real but also misremembered personal myth-making. It's a web of faith and science and myth, spinning itself around our bodies. Until we are so tangled we cannot tell where our bodies end and the myth begins.

Historian Hanne Blank notes in her book *Virgin* that anthropologists trace the evolution of virginity by the appearance of particular social factors. As fathers became the backbone of families and controlled access to goods and services, wealth and property began to be passed down through a patriarchal system. As such, knowing it was their genetic offspring they were protecting and providing for was a big deal. Virginity was key, as Blank observes: "Because virginity can render paternity knowable."[11]

Long before Mary gave birth, med-free in that barn, like a goddamn hippie, a system developed in which a woman could trade her virginity for access to material goods and protection for herself and her children. The downside was, as Blank explains, that "virginity lost before marriage often rendered the woman unmarriageable, useless on the marriage market."

Outdated as it is, the idea of virginity defining women's value still shapes our world. It's been the subject of fierce debate in Congress. Abstinence-only education was deemphasized in favor of a more comprehensive curriculum under Obama, but Donald Trump is once again incentivizing it with federal dollars, and it's still being pushed in over half the states in America.[12] According to a 2018 report from the Kaiser Family Foundation, thirty-seven states require that sex education, when taught at all, must include abstinence; twenty-six states require that abstinence be stressed.[13] All this despite study after study showing that a focus on abstinence does nothing to lower rates of STIs and pregnancies but, in fact, may increase them because it denies teens real information about protection, about their bodies, and about the realities of their lives.

Educational programs that teach abstinence make sex out to be something that defines you, for girls in particular. A common sex ed metaphor is the tape lesson. A piece of tape, representing a woman, is applied to a male student's arm and then is pulled off. Students see the skin and oil residue left on the tape and are told that is like sex. Eventually, that tape, if stuck to too many men, will lose its ability to bond. The lesson being, sex leaves you dirty and emotionally damaged.

It's a story I heard over and over as a child. Sex would break you. Sex would ruin you. And yet, sex was exactly the thing you were supposed to do once you were married. It's a confusing set of messages, not easy to reconcile. Sex is dirty up until the moment you exchange vows in a heterosexual union. And then, if there is a problem in your marriage, well, it must be because you're not having enough sex.

Given the sheer amount of mystery that still exists around the bodies of women and the process of birth, it would seem that the womb is truly the final frontier. A dark interiority that is loosely defined, the subject of mythologies we still teach in classrooms when we tell children that sex is dirty, sex ruins a woman, and virginity is a gift. These mythologies are born of male fear and a need for control. They lead to the veneration of virgins—Mary, yes, but also Saint Agatha, the patron saint of cockblocking, who was killed for the crime of refusing to sleep with men because she was so devoted to purity. Saint Agnes, who was dragged through the streets naked by an angry mob of men for making a vow of perpetual purity. Saint Lucy, who decided she'd rather be beheaded than sleep with her pagan husband. These women refused to put out, and we canonized them for it. We laud them for their ability to stay pure until death. For their commitment to virginity. These are the ideal women.

The other women we revere? Mothers. Sexual purity and motherhood are not mutually exclusive these days, but the vast majority of children are still conceived the old-fashioned way. Meaning, motherhood implies a lack of "purity." And yet, there is a moral expectation that mothers should project the idea of purity. A maternal appearance of perpetual virginity. One that radiates beauty, but not sexuality; that is maternal, but not earthy. One that pleases, but doesn't provoke. Which, of course, usually means white. *Pure* is not a label our society often bestows on black women. A 2018 study published in the *Psychology of Women Quarterly* found that black women are more likely to be sexualized and dehumanized than are white women.[14] In this way, the purity myth is a tool of white supremacy. If purity is moral capital, it's yet another kind of capital that women of color are disproportionately denied.

A maniacal obsession with purity can be all-consuming for women, who must always be vigilant for possible attacks and impropriety. "What to Wear When You Are 30?" "Modest Swimsuits for Mothers." "Office Appropriate Attire." Guide after guide advises women on how to influence how other people see and perceive them. A Facebook group for mothers I joined dedicates a whole subgroup to clothes, where members provide feedback on what is appropriate to wear for work, for parties, for outings with the family. Women walk around constantly afraid to smile, to wear low-cut shirts, for fear a man will get the wrong message from us, from our bodies. Imagine what women could do if they didn't have to worry about presenting themselves in a way that protected them from men, protected men from the mysteries of women's bodies. Imagine the autonomy.

The virginity myth allows a woman's sexuality to be defined by a man. It asks her to sublimate her own desires and frames desires that fall outside of heterosexual marriage between two cisgender people as deviant. In their 1972 pamphlet *The Power of Women and the Subversion of the Community*, which—remarkably or depressingly—still feels revolutionary, Mariarosa Dalla Costa and Selma James note that a woman's "childhood is a preparation for martyrdom: we are taught to derive happiness from clean sex on whiter than white sheets; to sacrifice sexuality and other creative activity at one and the same time."[15] Ending the myth of the vaginal orgasm, Costa and James argue, would end the idea that a woman's desires and pleasure were subject to the whims of the phallus. Reconnecting a woman with the power of her body is to reintegrate a woman with the possibility of her entire being.

In college, my purity ring got stuck on a shower loofah. When I extricated it, the leaves were bent. I put it away after that, joking with my friends about the implications of having broken this symbol of my virginity in the shower.

I did pull the ring back out on my honeymoon. Laughing, I gave it to my husband and told him the story. He put it away and I never saw it again.

We didn't have sex while we were dating. Abstinence was a mandate my husband took seriously and one I took seriously only because he did. Plus, I was hiding a secret. I was hiding the fact that I had gotten drunk in a dorm room with some boys. I believed I had been assaulted. I couldn't tell my boyfriend. To admit to that event would have compromised my virginity, compromised my desirability.

Once, in the early years of marriage, I was tempted to say something, to clear the air and unburden myself of a lapse I was beginning to think might not be entirely my fault. In bed one night, I asked my husband a hypothetical question: What if someone had been assaulted? What then?

He told me that he was happy I hadn't been. He wouldn't have married me if I hadn't been a virgin. He wouldn't have wanted me to be the mother of our children.

I said nothing. After all, maybe nothing had happened. I hadn't bled afterward. At the time, I believed what I'd been taught about the hymen, that it was a membrane sealing the vagina and that any dick entering or exiting would leave physical evidence of penetration.

When my husband was my fiancé, I had shown him articles that explained what the hymen really was and that described how it could be disrupted by any number of activities, that it was more of a myth about virginity than an actuality. But I only half-believed these articles myself. I was nervous. I didn't want him to hate me, to devalue me for what I might have lost—what might have been taken from me. It didn't occur to me until much later that by tying my value to my virginity, I had already allowed him to devalue me.

During the divorce, my ex claimed that I owed him money—$100,000—for the time and effort he put into developing and educating my mind. It was laughable. I laughed. My lawyer laughed. What a concept. It wasn't rooted in the law, she assured me. I had nothing to worry about. But we still had to talk about it in mediation, where the mediator pursed his lips and, in one thirty-minute closed-door meeting, got that number taken out of the settlement.

Afterward, that line item, my $100,000 brain, became a joke I told my friends. "Be nice to me. This brain is worth $100,000!"

But once, while sipping wine with a friend at dinner, my joke fell flat. "I don't like this," she said. "It's because you're only valued for your parts. How much was your virginity worth?"

This woman knew nothing of my sexual past. Of my fears and anxieties. And yet, she knew everything. She was trained as a sociologist and could see the systems and forces at play in the lives of women. Too often, we are all just holding on. Too often, it is too hard for us to lift our heads and see beyond our own suffering to the systemic issues.

In 2013, the *British Medical Journal* published a study that found that 0.08 percent of respondents believed they had had a virgin birth.[16] The story has been mocked online, the statistics questioned. But in an interview, one of the lead researchers, Amy Herring, professor of statistical science and research professor of global health at Duke University, certified that the findings were true. The survey was conducted anonymously via computer, and for whatever reason, forty-five respondents reported that their pregnancy had happened without intercourse.

It's a punchline of a statistic. Low-hanging fruit of a joke. These dumb women. These confused women. And maybe it's a mistake. And yet, I understand, in my gut, how they might hold that belief. The culture of virginity can be too strong and too hard to resist. What would I have said to my fiancé if that night I don't remember had resulted in a pregnancy? What would I have believed? It took me thirteen years to talk about the possibility of that moment. How would I have responded if confronted with proof of it just weeks later? How could I look down on other women who might be struggling with the trauma of assault and the deeply held belief that it would ruin them? Something like that can challenge your ideology, your entire worldview.

No, far easier to believe in miracles than the fact that your entire life is based on a lie. Far easier to believe that the life within you is born of wonder rather than that the men outside of you are trained to destroy you.

What do we expect to happen in a world where women are taught that their bodies are the ultimate gift and men are taught to take without recourse?

What does purity mean in a culture where the majority of women have been harassed, cat-called, and had unsolicited dicks sent to them in messages or thrust at them on the subway?[17] What can it mean when one in five women is sexually assaulted—and maybe that number is higher, but they won't or can't admit it, because to admit it would mean the loss of everything they are holding onto. The things that keep them alive.

I was married for twelve years, but I never once told my husband about that night in college. I barely told myself. How could I square my lived realities?

In her short story "The Blank Page," writer Karen Blixen, under the pen name Isak Dinesen, tells the story of the Convent of Veho, where aging nuns weave flax into the finest white sheets, which are used on the wedding nights of the princesses of Portugal. In the morning, the newly bloodstained sheets are cut up and sent to the convent, where they are framed and hung on a wall, with notes about the princess whose blood they showcase. Over the years, the princesses come to the convent to look at these offerings. But they spend most of their time looking at the single frame containing a blank sheet.

Dinesen's story is layered. It is told to a young couple by an old woman sitting at the gate of a city. "When a royal and gallant pen, in the moment of its highest inspiration, has written down its tale with the rarest ink of all—where, then, may one read a still deeper, sweeter, merrier and more cruel tale than that?" the old woman asks, before supplying the answer: "Upon the blank page."[18]

The story then is a story of absence rather than presence, of things done off the page that have been framed by the story of maidenhood. Its silence speaks of those moments and truths that can only be rendered by a white sheet. It's the story of virginity.

In 2018, eight months after I left my husband, I sat in my new bedroom watching the Kavanaugh hearings on my laptop. My phone vibrated with an endless stream of text messages from my friends, each one watching, each one going through her own realization—something like this had happened to her, to us. We had all been there in a room with a man. We had all come out changed. We had all forgotten, or had made ourselves forget, because we had no way of saying the truth and coming out alive.

"If I had told my parents," a friend texted, "I never would have been allowed to study abroad that next summer, I never would have been able to have some of the best experiences of my life." I thought about my own marriage, the one I ended. It wouldn't have existed if I had said what had happened. For each of us, our shame was born of what we had been told about our purity and the ways the purity myth had shaped our actual lived experience of womanhood. We can begin to loosen the stranglehold of patriarchal power on our bodies by rejecting this myth, both individually and culturally.

If I had told my fiancé what had happened, he wouldn't have believed that I was worth marrying. I knew that then. Now that knowledge is deeply upsetting, but at the time, as a girl raised to be pure and looking to find something, anything good to hold onto, it made sense. Even in 2005, even now, this makes sense to more women than we'd like to think.

He did look for blood in our honeymoon bed. Blood did eventually come in the form of a small lump of tissue, which made me question whether anything even happened in that dorm room. But I still didn't dare breathe a word. I knew better. For him, purity was as much a moral state as a physical one. What had happened in that dorm room, that night, was a blank sheet I would keep returning to, and it might always be.

These days, there is no pretending about my purity. I have two children. I will sleep with men on the first date or third, or whenever. I had been holding onto so many beliefs and expectations of my body for so long that I let them go the moment my marriage was over. I'm too tired to do anything less than what I want. In a way, what happens in those rooms, too, is a kind of white sheet. A freedom. A letting go.

Some interpretations of Dinesen's story read a queer story onto that blank sheet. Others point out the implicit racism of ascribing purity to whiteness. The narrative of purity, wherever it is found, is damaging. As Dinesen's story tells us, the limits of our stories are not the limits of our experiences. And our traumas are not the only things worth pinning to a wall.

Or maybe that's just me putting language where silence should exist.

After the divorce, I asked about the purity ring. *Where had it gone? Did he have it?*

No, he told me, it was lost. It had disappeared into the home we'd lived in for twelve years. Gone for good the day I left. I'll never look for it again.

Miscarriage

I gave birth to death one September.

I had been training for a half marathon and noticed my breasts felt tender as they jostled around on my runs. I took a pregnancy test. It was positive. I told my husband. I told my brother. I was excited. My oldest child was a year and a half at the time and an easy toddler—happy, a good sleeper. I wanted another. I wanted to give her a sibling. And because I'd had a healthy first pregnancy, and my doctor said I could, I kept running.

Two weeks later, I began to bleed. I noticed the blood on a day I worked from home. Just some spotting in my underwear. I wasn't sure what it meant, if it meant anything. Pregnancy makes weird vaginal secretions. A primordial soup of crotch slime—dissected and analyzed only on the deepest, darkest pregnancy message boards, where women post pictures and chime in on the "normal or not normal" debate.

Doctors don't tell you about the crotch slime. Nor do pregnancy books. I never read about it in even the most candid advice columns. But in those early days, wondering whether the fetus will live or die, and in the later days, too, waiting for the mucous plug to fall out and the water to break, expectant parents read their underwear like a fortune teller looking for life and death in tea leaves.

The spotting was light. But I frantically searched for answers—reading unreliable websites, blogs full of pseudoscientific speculation, mom forums—the gutters of internet worry. There was nowhere else to turn. I was too early for a doctor's appointment. I am a woman who has irregular periods, especially when I am running. I hadn't even noticed my period's absence until my breasts felt sore. If I hadn't taken the pregnancy test, maybe I would have thought it was just an unusually heavy period coming on.

Technology is both a blessing and a bind. Early detection gives pregnant people options and opportunities to choose whether to carry a pregnancy or not. But there are downsides, too. Pamela Geller, PhD, an associate clinical and health psychology professor at Drexel University in Philadelphia, believes that early screening heightens the grief over miscarriage.[1] Not all doctors agree on this; it's a hard thing to quantify. But it's clear that as advances in technology illuminate our interiority better, sooner, we project into these dark spaces more of our hopes and dreams and biases. Stripped of context, a pulsing mass of zygote is called a baby by some and a fetus by others. An estimated 10 to 30 percent of known pregnancies end in miscarriage. Pregnancy tests can give false positives. They can also test positive for chemical pregnancies, when the pregnancy loss occurs very early on, before implantation in the uterus is fully completed.

The first trimester is shadowed by death. From the moment a person knows they're pregnant, they know they can also miscarry. The fear never goes away. Not really. Most miscarriages happen in the first thirteen weeks. Past twenty weeks is considered the "safe zone" for announcing a pregnancy. But I know many women who didn't announce until they were about to deliver for fear of having to unannounce. Message boards and conversations are filled with fear, and, in an effort to hold it at bay, the small assurances of the life we cannot see but bear witness to: kick counts, heartbeats, ultrasounds, movement.

In the end, to carry a potential for life is to also carry a potential for death. You cannot separate the two.

I googled. I found evidence that suggested both that my pregnancy was safe and that it was not. But I knew. Or maybe I didn't actually "know"; maybe this was just the one time that my persistent sense of doom was right.

"I'm having a miscarriage," I told my husband that night.

"You're probably just overreacting," he said.

The next morning, the bleeding had stopped. But by the afternoon, it was back, and heavier. This time my stomach was cramping.

I called my doctor, who said to come in the next day. So, I put in a heavy pad. Made dinner. Said nothing to my husband. Put my daughter to bed. As I rocked her, I could feel the cramps roiling my stomach. My thighs felt damp. Later, I saw I had bled through the pad and onto my jeans. But in that moment, I held her sleeping body against me—head between my breasts, body curled against my stomach. Where she still fit. Where babies are designed to fit. And I sat there and felt her breath, watched the flush of her warm cheeks, touched the sweat of her sleepy hands, while life poured out of me and made me sticky with its reality.

When I put her down, I went downstairs, took some Tylenol, told my husband again I was miscarrying, told him I'd called the doctor.

"We'll see what the doctor says," he countered.

I said nothing but walked to the basement, the quiet, dark bathroom where I sat on the toilet and flushed what remained of a pregnancy away.

The next day, the doctor confirmed it. I'd had a miscarriage at about six weeks, or maybe seven or eight. Who could say, really, since my periods were so irregular.

When I came home and told my husband conclusively it had happened, he was upset. "I wish you hadn't been running so hard," he said. I didn't respond. I didn't probe his meaning. It felt clear: I had caused this.

To be capable of life is to also be capable of death.

In March 2019, lawmakers in Iowa attempted to pass a fetal personhood bill. The bill would have made it a crime—a felony—to kill a fetus, even if the fetus's existence was not known. The Iowa House refused to bring it to a vote after the state senate passed the bill with an added amendment that changed the wording from "terminates a human pregnancy" to "causes the death of an unborn person" and defined "unborn person" as the joined cells existing from "fertilization to live birth." It's a subtle shift in language but one that vastly changes the situation.

The fetal personhood movement is part of the pro-life agenda, which seeks to end access to abortion. Today, thirty-eight states and the federal government have fetal homicide laws that treat the fetus as a potential crime victim separate from the mother. Since the *Roe v. Wade* decision in 1973, there have been several hundred cases in which pregnant women were prosecuted and convicted under fetal personhood laws. Their crimes include getting into a car accident that resulted in the death of their fetus, miscarrying, and delivering stillborn babies.

In 2013, Purvi Patel was convicted of feticide and neglect of a dependent after she experienced a miscarriage. Patel went to St. Joseph's Hospital in Mishawaka, Indiana, bleeding and in pain. She had miscarried and had left the fetal remains in a trash bin. Authorities arrested her at the hospital for "neglect of a dependent" and later added the "feticide" charge after they found text messages between Patel and a friend that allegedly indicated Patel was trying to induce a miscarriage. Patel was convicted, though her conviction was overturned on appeal.[2]

Patel and other women like her—typically, those targeted for prosecution are low-income and women of color—are not a danger to their families or society at large. But they serve jail time as criminals for delivering death instead of life. Even when they don't go to jail, or their convictions are overturned on appeal, they often suffer the wide-ranging mental, emotional, and financial costs of facing charges over a stillbirth that undermine their lives and well-being. Not to mention the other women who see this and internalize it as a warning, a lesson about the value of their lives versus the lives they are carrying or may someday carry.

Recent studies have shown that, in fact, many human pregnancies end in miscarriage, typically very early in pregnancy, before the pregnancy is known or even suspected.[3] There are various causes for these miscarriages: perhaps a chromosomal abnormality in the baby, perhaps the pregnancy wasn't viable, perhaps there was a problem with the cervix or the uterus. Rarely is it stress or alcohol or even drugs.

Few women know this. In fact, study after study shows that miscarriages are shrouded in feelings of secrecy, shame, and guilt. A 2015 study found that most women erroneously believed that miscarriage was rare and, of women who had had miscarriages, 47 percent felt guilty, 41 percent reported feeling that they had done something wrong, 41 percent felt alone, and 28 percent felt ashamed.[4]

The pro-life movement wants them to feel this way. We live in a culture that wants to limit women's reproductive rights and that restricts access to healthcare, yet blames a woman when her body does exactly what it needs to when rejecting a nonviable fetus.

We pass laws that criminalize women for miscarriages that even doctors don't know how to prevent.

Miscarriage. Stillbirth. Even when medical evidence suggests these losses were inevitable, their weight falls on the mothers' shoulders and is expected to leave indelible marks on their hearts. In her 1980 book *Mother Love*, Elisabeth Badinter writes of the death of a child: "The fact that [the mother] can give birth to another child nine months later does not cancel the effect of the death. For the intangible worth we ascribe to each human being, including the viable fetus, no tangible substitute exists."[5]

The enterprise of life has always come with the threat of death. Birth is dangerous for both pregnant people and their babies. Miscarriage and stillbirths are an ever-present reality. Advancements in technology have dramatically improved the odds of survival, giving many of us healthier, longer lives. But with these developments has come the illusion of control. That in some way we can prevent death. Or criminalize its causes.

For almost all of human history, death was a way of life. Especially for babies and small children. Parents often didn't attend the burials of their infants, who were usually buried unnamed. As Badinter notes, "Given the high infant mortality rate that existed until the end of the eighteenth century, if the mother had developed an intense attachment to each of her newborn babies, she certainly would have died of sorrow." Badinter points to the example of a mother in an English lying-in hospital who, after watching two young children die, observed that she still had a lot more children inside of her.

Even in nineteenth-century America, babies who survived into childhood often fell victim to diseases like yellow fever and tuberculosis, which wiped out entire communities. Death was so common as to be woven into the narratives of childhood. In the popular antebellum children's book *The Tragi-Comic History of the Burial of Cock Robin with the Lamentation of Jenny Wren*, Jenny

Wren arranges a funeral for Cock Robin. The book teaches children about death, funeral rites, and the etiquette of grief. A Sunday school tract titled "Heaven," published in the 1850s, prepared children for death by depicting a conversation between a mother and son. "Is it not dreadful to die?" asks the boy. "Is it not dreadful to such as love God and do all they can to serve and please him?" answers the mother.

Everything changed in the twentieth century. Sanitation and vaccinations meant that fewer children died. And during the Industrial Revolution the concept of the home was invented. In agricultural societies, women had worked alongside men, as did their children. Work and home were not separate realms, because both happened in the same space. Factory work upended that arrangement.

Initially, many women as well as men worked in factories, leaving their infants at home in the care of older siblings, other relatives, or hired help. Working conditions in the factories were horrible, and the physical demands exhausting. Popular humanitarian efforts led by white suffragists and Christian crusaders worked to get women and children out of factories and into the home, and in 1903, the Supreme Court upheld an Oregon law that prohibited women from working a ten-hour day. The law was an example of benevolent sexism: protecting women from long hours on the basis of the belief that women were more delicate than men.[6] It appeared to be a noble enterprise, aiding women who were being exploited for wage labor. And it may have looked like liberation at the time—a woman, tasked with the care of children and the economic burden of a home and a life, was then told, "You don't have to work anymore; you just have to care for your family."

But in reality, this freedom was just another cage. Keeping women out of factories transitioned them from poorly paid manual labor to unpaid domestic labor, while ensuring men had less competition for factory jobs. It's a great trick of American society: tell people you're setting them free while stripping them of their freedoms. Of course, even then, many working-class women didn't have a choice as to whether or not they worked outside the home.

A pregnancy guide originally published in 1912 reflected these evolving social mores, advising women: "No single influence is more unfavorable to comfort and health during pregnancy than is idleness, so that every prospective should occupy herself with congenial work and fitting diversions. The kind of occupation makes no essential difference, so long as it does not overtire either the body or the mind."[7] The book acknowledges that some women have to work. But it urges them not to work too hard. Ergo, the book tells them, the only work that is suitable for a good mother is domestic work.

Employers used to refuse to employ married women, especially in white-collar, respectable industries like banking and insurance. In 1932, the Economic Act prohibited more than one person in a household from holding a government job, forcing many women to lose their jobs, sending them back home.

These laws disproportionately affected black families, who have historically been more likely to be two-income households as a result of a racial wealth gap caused by generations of exploitation and discriminatory wages and hiring practices. Claudia Goldin, professor of economics at Harvard University and director of the Development of the American Economy program at the National Bureau of Economic Research, notes in her paper "Female Labor Force Participation: The Origin of Black and White Differences, 1870 and 1880," that since 1880, 35.4 percent of married black women and 73.3 percent of single black women were in the labor force compared with 7.3 percent of married white women and 23.8 percent of single white women.[8] Both before and after marriage, more white women could opt out of the workforce, while black women remained in.

The women who did leave the workforce often joined an invisible workforce. In "The Power of Women and the Subversion of the Community," Mariarosa Dalla Costa and Selma James write, "Woman . . . has been isolated in the home, forced to carry out work that is considered unskilled, the work of giving birth to, raising, disciplining, and servicing the worker for production."[9] This labor was glorified, as exemplified by the image of the mother as the angel of the house.

As the concept of home became clearer, women became smaller. For smart, ambitious women with no outlet for their skills except their children, motherhood and homemaking became all-consuming identities. Dalla Costa and James write that women decorate their homes because their homes are the only proof they exist. The same logic could be used for pouring one's life into children. Children become a woman's reason for being, her proof of existence. As if her own existence weren't enough.

Rousseau preached in his influential philosophical text *Emile* that if society was to return to its natural order, mothers must return to being mothers. A good society began with mothers at home raising children. Their bodies were conduits of social order.

For American society—in the early twentieth century as now—unemployed men are a crisis, but unemployed women are mothers. Trapped in the home, women's attention turned toward the care and well-being of their children in a way it never had before. And from there, every new advancement in labor-saving devices led to increased pressure on mothers to perform motherhood.

Through these concurrent advances in science and technology, American childhood became what it is today. Our children survive to adulthood at rates unimaginable to our foremothers. They are protected from cruel working conditions, surrounded by love and care.

Modern childhood was born then. Modern motherhood was, too.

In 2015, I was a mother of two small children and also worked as a writer. I worked out of my house, I worked whenever I could. Sometimes I woke up at four in the morning to sneak in writing time. Other times, I stayed up until two. During the day, I cared for my kids. They didn't nap well. So, I read in stolen moments while they played with playdough. I answered email on the playground.

Once, as I tapped out an email while my kids dug in the sand, I overheard a mother say to her friend how smartphones are making us bad parents. I wanted to throw my phone at her head and remind her that Ma Ingalls lost Carrie in a field while she did laundry by hand. I said nothing, as is the Midwestern way, just quietly seethed with a mixture of rage and guilt.

Google "mommy put down the iPhone" and you'll get millions of hits, the top ones being articles like these:

"Mommy put down your iPhone and Look at Me!"

"How I Put Down the iPhone and Started Being a Mom"

"Dear mom on the iPhone: Let me tell you what you don't see"

Before the iPhone, it was a washer and dryer, a dishwasher, a microwave, a refrigerator—items optimized to make domestic life easier but stirring up unease about how women should spend all that free time. Around the turn of the nineteenth century, there was an explosion of literature from doctors and scientists about parenting, including G. Stanley Hall's *Adolescence* and L. Emmett Holt's *The Care and Feeding of Children*. The Children's Bureau was established in 1912, the sole purpose of which was to ensure the care and well-being of America's children. According to the Oxford English Dictionary, the term "parenting" was first used in 1918 and exploded in popularity in the 1970s when experts like Dr. Spock and Bruno Bettelheim jumped into the mix of parenting experts.

Under the guise of science, parenting became a full-time job. Studies showed parents (primarily women then and now) how to care for their children, how long to breastfeed, when to give babies cow's milk, how to place the baby in the crib—no, wait, now you co-sleep—no, wait, let the baby cry it out. But how dare you let the baby cry without going to comfort them, how could you? Don't you know studies prove this harms babies? Except wait, maybe they don't. Or maybe we're confused. We are definitely confused.

Parenting in this age of science and pseudoscience means sifting through contradictory car seat recommendations, crib warnings, stroller warnings, advice columns, studies, and justifications for everything.

Today's technology, like smartphones and the internet, allows mothers to order groceries, set hair appointments, see test results, read grade transcripts, and do their actual paid work all from their home. But it also comes with increased expectations of overattentiveness to their child's life. Because "the machine doesn't exist that makes and minds children," write Della Costa and James, so a mother "is always on duty."[10] Where once a mother had household work, she now has childcare—a constant supervision of every poop, cough, fart, panting, sound, fingernail, heartbeat.

You think I'm kidding? I was sent home from the hospital with both of my newborns with a sheet to mark every feeding, every wet diaper, every shit. The idea was to fill out the form for the first six weeks of the child's life, or even longer. I filled it out religiously with my first child. The sheet was a mess of scrawled midnight notes in pencil or lip liner. With modern technology, parents can track a baby's sleep and poop cycles in apps and can watch their infant sleep with the hypervigilance of an elite spy operation—3-D imaging and body heat sensors. And if we *can* do these things, it follows, then, of course, we should, we must.

These expectations not only control a mother's time but also how she thinks and how she acts.

There's a scene in the CBS show *Criminal Minds* in which JJ, a pregnant FBI profiler, halts a conversation about a killer to put headphones over her pregnant belly. She tells the others she doesn't want her child to hear the gory details of the conversation, as if talk of dismembered women will permanently scar the developing fetus still inside of her. The rest of the team of analytical thinkers readily assents, no questions asked.

The barrier between mother and child is physically permeable and philosophically up for debate. A uniting experience of American pregnancy is receiving the list of things you're forbidden from putting in your body so as not to harm your fetus: alcohol, caffeine, medication, lunch meat, and much more. It's true that what the mother ingests will reach the fetus, even if the risk to the fetus isn't always clear. Other links between mother and baby slip into a nearly spiritual realm. Just as fetal cells cross the placenta and enter the mother's bloodstream, remaining forever lodged somewhere inside her, mothers, too, leave their cells in their children: these cells cross the placenta in the opposite direction, strengthening the immune system and, well—no one is quite sure what else.

The science leads easily to superstition. Today, a thriving contemporary market of goods exists to promote fetal positivity and protect your baby from the wicked influences of the world. Bellybuds, a $49.99 sound system for your unborn baby, advertises its ability to make a positive maternal impression by transmitting sound into the womb through the belly. Rival company Babypod argues that mothers need to insert a tampon-like speaker in their vagina to be sure the music reaches the baby.

The logic is ancient. Upset the mother and ruin the baby; if the mother is sweet, the child will be sweet too. It's a logic rooted in biological fact—the state of a pregnant person's body, from basic physical health to emotional well-being, does affect their fetus to some degree—that has been twisted into an equally powerful psychological fiction: the idea that what a pregnant woman sees and thinks about will manifest in her unborn child dates back centuries, and persists today.

In 1897, C. J. Bayer wrote a pleading appeal to pregnant women in his book *Maternal Impressions*:

> That a mother who is in the condition to which attention is called, who has an imperfectly formed object, such as a monstrosity of any kind in her mind, and who dwells upon it, or who has impure or vulgar thoughts and mean or unholy ideas, or who has murder in mind—that is, would like to kill her unborn babe—will impress such a formation of the brain structure of her offspring, as will form its desires in the direction which her thoughts have taken.[11]

A 1919 public health education poster scoffs at the idea of maternal impression, but then still advises women to be emotionally on guard for their baby's safety: "Worry, fear and anger may affect his mothers' blood, which supplies his food. Therefore, she should be calm, happy and sweet-tempered."

"Be sweet!" is still the dominant advice given to pregnant women today. Take a rest. Sit down. Don't worry your pregnant mind. Think of the baby. Mothers are advised not to be stressed out. Studies on pregnant woman do show links between increases in maternal stress and fetal stress, and maternal stress has even been linked to preterm birth and schizophrenia. There is also a potential link between stress and lower birth weight.[12] But we routinely overlook the culture and system that overworks women physically and mentally, that is so powerfully bigoted and un-just that day-to-day life here can be a potentially deadly stressor for members of marginalized groups, and instead we place the blame and the burden of stress on the mother.[13] Pregnant women who expose themselves to that which is not sweet—a sip of wine, some cold medicine, or a gory crime police procedural before bed—they are selfish. They take no heed of maternal impressions and do not put their child's needs before their own.

Science has historically believed that women's bodies are per-meable vessels: weak clay to the man's molded steel. Pregnant bodies, even more so. There is a bias at play even when the facts are unknown or neutral: in a recent interview with NPR, Janet Williams, a professor of pediatrics at the University of Texas Health Science Center in San Antonio, advised women that there are too many unknowns with drinking even a little while pregnant, so women should just avoid it altogether, which is both an understandable suggestion from someone who wants to avoid a lawsuit and yet also completely regressive.[14]

If a pregnant woman were to avoid all unknowns, she would be locked in a quiet closet listening only to Mozart—and mom blogs would still debate how harmful the light coming in from the crack under the door is. And how selfish she is for not being more in shape.

Chained to a child or chained to a desk, a woman's value is contained within her (re)productive abilities. And when those abilities fail, through miscarriage, stillbirth, medical problems, infertility, or she opts out of the whole process, we don't know how to see her. We can't see her.

I once interviewed Alyssa Mastromonaco, the White House deputy chief of staff for operations under the Obama administra-tion, for a story I was writing about her book, *So Here's the Thing*. During our conversation, I asked her how hard it was to write about choosing not to be a mother. "It's all people want to talk about," she said.

I laughed. "When you have kids, it's still the same."

"Fucked either way," said Mastromonaco.

I think about that a lot. *Fucked either way.* Mother or not mother. Pregnant or not, our life is defined by the reproductive role we're expected to play.

I thought I was responsible for my miscarriage. Had my running destroyed the baby? The thought lay in the back of my mind. Even though I knew better, knew that miscarriages could just happen. They were common. And yet . . . and yet. My husband voiced it, too.

The evening he did, I couldn't sleep. I spent all night in the office, crying and frantically googling whether running could cause a miscarriage. Don't do that, by the way. The result was a clotted mess of stories on message boards and fearmongering pieces from websites trying to get traffic from anxiety clicks like mine.

I run for so many reasons. Health, fitness, vanity—sure. But I also do it to remind myself I am a body. After giving birth, each heavy step, each quivering muscle reminded me that this body did not belong to a child, did not belong to a man, who made demands of it. It belongs to me. Each pain. Each triumph. This body was mine. Mine. Each quiver of skin. Mine. I alone could feel its pain. I alone could feel its strength.

That night of anxiety searching, I wanted to exculpate myself. I wanted to know that it was okay to run. That it was okay to be an independent body. I did not get that assurance from the internet. I did not get that assurance from my husband. I did not get that assurance from my doctor, who just hedged and said I was probably fine and these things happen. I didn't get that assurance from all the studies I read about running and pregnancy and fitness.

In the end, I ran the race. My husband wasn't there. He didn't bring our daughter. Instead, I ran it with my friend Megan. But when I crossed that finish line, it was just me—all of me.

There is a connection between mother and child, one that holds fast even into the child's adulthood. The subcortical region of our brain is deeply influenced by this first love, this longest-lasting connection. But the extent of it remains unknown. No one can say for sure whether the fact that I watched crime shows while pregnant will make my children deviants or allergy medicine taken out of desperation in the second trimester will be the reason my daughter doesn't make it into Yale. No one can say whether my running caused a miscarriage or my love of Sonic hamburgers hurt my children's cholesterol. But no one can tell me that my running isn't why my children are also incredible, strong, and competitive, either. No one can tell me that those books I read out loud to them in the womb aren't the reason they are innovative thinkers, good with words, excellent at puns.

The legend of La Llorona, in Mexican folklore, is the story of a woman who drowns her children in a rage after her husband leaves her for another woman. She is a woman scorned, and to punish her husband, she turned life into death. La Llorona is cursed to walk the rivers weeping, seeking the souls of her children. She cannot find them, so she grabs the children of other women and pulls them into the water.

In *Women Who Run with the Wolves*, Dr. Clarissa Pinkola Estés relates another story of La Llorona, told to her by a ten-year-old boy. In this version of the story, the mother loses her children because they are poisoned by water from the river that has been polluted by the factory the mother works for. The children's death is not her fault, not truly. Yet she is still cursed to stand by the river and weep. She still pays with her soul for something beyond her control.

In our stories, mothers whose children die, no matter why, even before they are born, are murderers. A woman who has a miscarriage or abortion or stillborn child is seen as fundamentally abhorrent. She is cursed. She has transgressed. She has failed in her most essential duty.

In March 2019, Texas lawmakers proposed a bill that would criminalize abortion and make it possible for women to receive the death penalty for having an abortion. Representative Tony Tinderholt, the Republican state legislator who introduced the bill, said it would make people "consider the repercussions" of having sex.[15]

He didn't mean people. He meant women. He meant women need to give birth or die. He meant that a body capable of life must give life. Should never need any other alternative.

It never occurred to me, until I began to run again a year after our second child was born, that I should have been angry when my husband blamed me for the miscarriage. He blamed my running. Blamed my body. Blamed my choices. But how could I be mad at him when I blamed me too? I blamed myself for choosing to run. For putting my own well-being over that of my child.

How soon we learn to sacrifice our bodies for the bodies of our children. As if our bodies and the lives within us were doomed to be at odds. But nature tells a different story.

Braided in our bodies are both life and death. Perhaps instead of an anomaly, this too is part of nature.

Part II

SECOND TRIMESTER

Congratulations, your baby is the size of a strawberry. A ripe red fruit, floating inside you. A foreign object. How quickly you learn to separate your sense of your baby from yourself. Your baby is a blueberry, a kumquat, a tiny gourd. A little bitty peanut. A bundle of pink or blue.

In the second trimester, it's time to sleep on your side or else you'll kill your baby. Fuck your comfort. You should also get the nursery perfect. Make it pristine. Spend a lot of money on this room in which your baby will refuse to sleep for the first year or five. But, of course, be careful of lifting heavy objects or inhaling paint fumes—you could kill your baby.

Plan a babymoon to ease the fragile ego of your husband, who will inevitably get pissy once the baby is born because he will feel cast aside. Remember it's your job to alleviate his uncomfortable feelings and care for your child. Have sex with him. Make him feel sexy. What about you? You're such a selfish bitch for asking. Better learn now how to juggle the labor of motherhood and the fragile ego of man.

Wait, you're married to a woman? You aren't married at all? Too bad. Get ready for the father jokes regardless. Having a baby is like experiencing all the biases of our culture in their most condensed and obvious form. Good luck.

This is also the perfect time to practice some self-care. Get a manicure, but worry about the toxins in nail polish. Get a haircut, but worry about inhaling fumes in the salon. Get a massage, but worry about how it can mess up your baby.

Your baby who is now a kiwi.

Your baby who is now a dragonfruit.

Your baby who is now a tiny, weird, albino squirrel floating in front of you like a ghost on a screen.

"Look, it's a boy!"

"You're having a girl!"

Your lab tech will tell you this, and you will have feelings about that announcement. Perhaps a boy, to you, means fewer hormones and feelings. Perhaps a girl, to you, means redemption. Perhaps it means bows. Perhaps it means baseball.

Your baby is a mango. Your baby is a baseball. Your baby is a tutu.

Your baby is not you.

You will begin to get the room ready, in pinks or blues. Or maybe you are woke and will choose grays, yellows, oranges. But it doesn't matter. People will shower you in gender-conforming clothes and the weight of gendered expectations for this little beefsteak tomato inside you. Time to think of footballs and ballet shoes and all the trappings of gender for your baby, who even before they are born is expected to perform. These expectations are to be, well, expected. If you don't foist them on this tiny papaya now, you will be considered weird and difficult. You don't want to be one of those difficult moms, do you? You know, the ones who get written about in viral news stories, where all the kids have long hair and gender-neutral names and the mother is a vegan homeschooler who birthed in a river. You don't want to be like that, right?

But that's also a performance. Learn now that you cannot win. Learn now that no matter what kind of mother you are, you will still be one of *those* moms. Wine mom. Cool mom. Tiger mom. You will be mocked. Something is wrong with what you are doing. I don't know what yet, but give it time. You are doing something wrong.

But for now, enjoy the zucchini inside you.

Hunger

All I wanted was a turkey sandwich—a thick cut of deli turkey heaped on seeded rye, one layer of crisp lettuce, then a tomato with a bit of salt, mayonnaise on both sides of the bread, a smear of spicy brown mustard on just one, and a thick, sliced kosher dill pickle on the other side. My body craved this sandwich every day once the constant motion in my stomach ceased and I no longer spent the mornings lying with my face on the cool tile of the bathroom floor hoping that the nausea would pass.

The sandwich just came to me, unbidden. I had never really had a sandwich like this. Not with this specificity. Down to the two gentle shakes of salt on the tomato. The lettuce, too, I'd choose carefully: iceberg lettuce, cool and crisp. Complementing the gentle weight of the tomato.

And the tomatoes, I wanted them to be from the farmer's market. The heavy, mottled kind, their skins bursting just a little. Warm, with streaks of green and brown.

I ate the sandwich at night, right before bed. I would put my daughter to bed and then walk heavily down the stairs, passing my husband, who sat watching *Star Trek* on the couch, on my way to the kitchen. He never participated in my ritual.

At my prenatal appointments, my doctor frowned at my weight. "What are you eating?" she asked. I shrugged.

"When I was pregnant with my son, I drank a lot of McDonald's shakes. I knew I shouldn't. But I couldn't stop," she said.

I smiled one of those "fuck you" kind of a smiles. You get good at those when you're pregnant.

I weighed close to two hundred pounds. My pre-pregnancy weight had been one-fifty. And that was up twenty pounds since the birth of my daughter. My relationship with my body size was complex. Eating, for a woman, is a fraught enterprise. We learn from an early age that smaller bodies are supposed to be better bodies. We ask for salads over anemic sandwiches, knowing that our worth lies in the ebb and flow of the skin around our waists. A whole industry has emerged to make us feel bad about food. We should cook it longer, slower, or not at all. It should be green and meatless. It should be full of protein and carbless. But no, wait, carbs are fine, we just can't have sugars. Except you can eat fruit, just not that fruit. Not eating is equated with restraint, with virtue. Eating is a luxury only the thin are allowed. A woman can eat if her body bears no evidence of it afterward.

When was the last time you enjoyed a meal without compunction, without restraint? Without guilt? For me, it was that sandwich.

"Losing the weight will be hard," my doctor added.

What I didn't say was, "Fuck you." What I didn't say was, "I was hungry." I was happy. That that sandwich was everything. And that once my child was born my pretext for profligate consumption of calories would go away and I'd be left again with salads and waters and tight-lipped "no, thank you, I would not like dessert" lies.

Instead, I said nothing. I went home and ate another sandwich.

At her first prenatal appointment, every pregnant woman in America is given a list of unsafe foods. These include coffee, soft cheese, raw fish, and deli meat. The list is a warning about foods that could harbor listeria or salmonella or high mercury levels. All bad for the baby. Or so the logic goes. Also, another guideline states how much a woman should gain during pregnancy: twenty to thirty pounds. A myriad of government agencies and groups create these rules, from the Environmental Protection Agency and the Food and Drug Administration to the Centers for Disease Control and Prevention and the American College of Obstetricians and Gynecologists.

In more ways than one, if you believed the doctors and several government agencies, my sandwich was poison.

For pregnant women, the grit, gristle, pleasure of our every bite is complicated by motherhood. When I was visibly pregnant, I had supermarket clerks ask me if I thought it was a good idea to buy the salmon in my cart. A Starbucks barista asked me whether my coffee should be decaf. When I said, "No, please give me the caffeine," she frowned and asked, "Is that wise?"

Family members looked askance when I ate Caesar dressing, suggesting I should be worried about the possibility of raw eggs. "Really?" I said. "It's bottled, on a shelf at Target."

Just be safe, they said.

Just think of the baby, they said.

As if the baby wasn't the only thing I thought of. As if the baby hadn't taken over my whole body. As if everything I thought I knew about the vast sea of my skin wasn't now completely foreign. Stretching, pulling, aching in ways I had never known.

As if I could stop thinking about the baby, whose presence leaked into my dreams—my subconscious imagining that I had left the baby in the grocery store, in a cupboard, in a drawer.

Even my earlobes looked thick with baby. How could I not think about the baby?

And behind each warning about safety lurked the other warning about weight. "Are you sure you aren't having twins?" a relative asked during both of my pregnancies.

The second time, with my second pregnancy, when I was more tired and cared less, I told her, "No, I'm just fat." And she laughed nervously, because I had said the thing we weren't supposed to say. That I looked like the little girl who chewed the stolen gum in the chocolate factory and Oompa Loompas were going to have to roll me away.

Once, when I asked my husband if he could help me off the couch, he mentioned he might need a giant spatula. And it was my turn to laugh then, because I was too tired for a fight. So tired from so many people pointing out the circumference of my body that, sure, what was another?

Other women, however, have found the experience of eating while pregnant freeing. A neighbor of mine, a mother of four, related with fondness how pregnancy was the first time in her life that she was seen not as fat, but as full of life. That gave her a chance to enjoy the food she put in her mouth instead of feeling scrutinized. For women who are seen as overweight, the freedom of eating while pregnant can be empowering. The food finds a righteous cause in the nourishment of the child. Food for the baby inside is good. Food just for the mother? To indulge or to withhold, that is the truly monstrous question.

In moments of extreme gender performance, women are allowed to be versions of themselves they would not otherwise be allowed to be. Brides can be demanding. Pregnant women can eat.

These moments of freedom are fleeting. Brides must become good wives. Pregnant women must eventually lose the weight.

And, of course, these liberations have their own limits. Brides can demand, but not so much that they turn into Bridezilla. Pregnant women are allowed to eat, just not too much or the "wrong" foods.

But which foods are appropriate and safe is more complicated and variable than the doctor's list makes it seem. In southeastern Nigeria, some pregnant women avoid eating snail to prevent their children from being sluggish.[1] Semai horticulturalists in Malaysia avoid eating unripe fruit because they believe it causes malaria. In Fiji, food taboos for pregnant women target specific forms of marine life believed to harm the fetus. In China, pregnant women avoid cooling foods, like watermelon, because these are thought to upset the balance of the pregnant woman's body.[2] Perhaps our food restrictions protect us from potentially unsafe foods. But that can't be the whole story because our cravings and our regulations are clearly culturally influenced. After all, pregnant women in Japan eat sushi. It would be nice to think that our medical advice is based purely on scientific data. But the truth is, cultural biases and assumptions are endemic in all aspects of medicine.

Emily Oster's book *Expecting Better* pushed back against US myths about what pregnant women should and should not do with the factual approach of an economist. Untangling correlation and causality, Oster digs deep into the scientific studies that inform the guidelines of the FDA, CDC, EPA, and American College of Obstetricians and Gynecologists that doctors draw on for advice. She concludes that most of the accepted wisdom regarding pregnancy isn't founded in science. For example, many doctors recommend that women avoid caffeine during pregnancy because studies done on mice and rats show a causal link between miscarriage and caffeine consumption. But, as Oster explains, to produce a miscarriage in rats, researchers had to pump them full of 250 milligrams of caffeine per day. Scaled up to human proportions, that's the equivalent of over sixty cups of coffee. Randomized controlled studies in humans face other difficulties. Namely, the woman's desire to drink coffee. Oster points out the link between an increase in nausea during pregnancy and carrying a baby to full term. Given that a nauseated pregnant person is less likely to want caffeine, studies may be reflecting the finding that women who weren't nauseated and therefore who did drink caffeinated coffee had more miscarriages than the women who didn't drink coffee (because they were nauseous as all hell).[3]

Oster's book recommends that women eat and drink what they like in moderation, noting that all too often the touted risks of a food or drink outweigh the evidence of that risk. But since Oster's book was published in 2013, I've yet to see a change in the way modern medicine polices the eating and drinking of mothers.

Of course, the lists telling women to avoid caffeine and sushi and lunchmeat and so many other things are about more than just the malingering mythologies of medicine. Ethnographers suggest that food taboos help regulate the process of life events, imbuing them with meaning and ritual. Foods desired and foods restricted make a liturgy for the process of our bodies. But why must it be a restriction of food? Why not a feast?

By restricting eating, patriarchy exerts a moderating influence on the process of life. All human life flows through a female body. And yet that body is not controlled by woman but is controlled by culturally defined and repressed expressions of who and what a woman, a mother, ought to be.

The rules, then, are less about science and more about how we culturally connect the embodiment of pregnancy to the world. How we order and make sense of our new bodies in this space. The rules are a liturgy of life. They are the language we hold onto—the guiding myths that give us meaning and order, as our bodies take on a new shape.

Research suggests that pregnancy cravings could be connected to hormones.[4] Some studies indicate that pregnancy cravings reveal actual dietary needs.[5] It's hard to know the truth. They could also be cultural. Certainly, our cravings are culturally defined. Women in Tennessee often crave fast food and sweets,[6] whereas women in Tanzania are more likely to crave meat, mangos, and yogurt.[7]

I love the lists of the things women have craved. On Reddit, women revealed that they wanted the following foods:[8]

Baked beans on vanilla ice cream

Spaghetti sandwiches on bread with mayo and garlic salt

Snickers wrapped in bacon

Tums

Raw red meat

Tuna salad on waffles

Each item a story of lack and of fullness. Of want and of withholding.

And do you indulge or do you hold back? Do you for once engage your most primal desires or do you restrain yourself? What a radical thing it would be to let women eat. To let women fill their hunger. And oh, the things we would eat!

Because pregnancy exists in the dissonant space between internal and external, our myths and misunderstandings about the relation between the body of the mother and the health of the baby deal not just with food but also with how mothers dress themselves and what media they consume.

In a Baby Center forum post from 2012, a woman, pregnant and in her first trimester, asks if she can cross her legs.[9] "I have heard this numerous times from my ma in law and also from my colleague that pregnant women should not sit cross legged. I find it extremely comfortable sitting with my legs crossed and feel that it sometimes takes the pain off my back." The woman says she's asked her doctor about it, who says crossing her legs is fine. But our culture around pregnancy trains us to be wary of risk, real or perceived, so she remains unsure. She asks the internet to answer.

The post has eleven responses, all debating the merits of crossing or not crossing your legs during pregnancy. Everyone has heard something about something from someone. They all believe they have the right answer.

The popular pregnancy website Ask Doctor Sears weighed in on the controversy, recommending that pregnant women keep their legs firmly planted on the floor.[10] Keeping your legs open, the site advises, keeps your blood pressure lower and aids in a smooth birth. Several studies suggest that crossing the legs at the knee increases blood pressure during testing.[11] But that's true for everyone, not just pregnant women.

The focus on mothers and the openness or closedness of their bodies has a long history that finds its roots in ideas about the morality and immorality of external bodily expression—of a mother and of her child.

Renaissance surgeon Ambroise Paré wrote in *On Monsters and Marvels* that a woman who crossed her legs too tightly would deform her baby. Similarly, a woman who bound her waist too tightly could turn her baby into a monster through her vanity.

This idea persisted through the Age of Enlightenment to the Victorian era, when in 1889 the *Rational Dress Society Gazette* argued, "In many cases the cripple, the idiot, the inebriate, the profligate, would find that they owed their sufferings and their sorrows to the folly of their mothers. Tight-laced women bequeath to their children an imperfect vitality, which often leads to vicious ways."[12]

Corsets, Victorian scolds noted, served only fashion and vanity. And what kind of mother would sacrifice the safety of her child in order to look good? It's very possible that tightly laced corsets did harm the reproductive organs of women. Just as it's possible that crossing our legs at the knees raises our blood pressure. It's also hard to parse out the answers, because doctors' advice regarding the corset was tightly bound to their ideas of appropriate morality for women, especially mothers.

In *The Corset: A Cultural History*, Valerie Steele cites medical texts that blame the corset for insanity, corruption of the blood, and horniness. One such scold is Orson Fowler, who pleaded in his 1846 *The Intemperance and Tight Lacing of the Corset* for women to "Unloose your corset . . . and remember that you are born, not to court and please, not to be courted and pleased by, fashionable rowdies, but to become wives and mothers."[13]

It's not that different from advice you might hear now. Forget fashion, ladies, you are not a sexual object. You are a wife. You are a mother. As if wives and mothers aren't sexual objects at all but merely wombs.

In 2018, Kate Middleton caused a stir by appearing in high heels in her third trimester. Commenters expressed worry about her safety, gently scolding her for prioritizing fashion over the life of her baby. This wasn't the first time the Duchess of Cambridge was concern-trolled about a fashion choice. In 2013, during her first pregnancy, her heel got caught on a grate in the street. A *Daily Mail* article cites numerous doctors proclaiming that wearing high heels during pregnancy is dangerous because a woman might fall. "Your center of gravity will be constantly changing," notes a doctor in an ABC News article about the controversy.[14]

Each article reminds mothers to put their child first. Reading those articles, it's not hard to hear the echoes of history— "remember that you were born . . . to become wives and mothers."

As far back as the ancient world, men could be found expressing fears over what a woman eats, wears, or thinks. Hippocrates,
in the fourth century BCE: "If a pregnant woman feels the desire
to eat earth or charcoal and then eats them, the child will show
signs of these things." Aristotle, in his humbly titled *Masterpiece*,
wrote that an adulteress having sex with her lover could conceive
of a child who looks like her husband by simply imagining his
face during conception. He added, "And through this power of
imaginative faculty it was that a woman, at the time of conception, beholding the picture of a black-a-moor, conceived and
brought forth a child, resembling an Ethiopian."[15]

A recurring legend of dubious historical documentation has
Hippocrates using this logic to save a princess accused of adultery
because she had given birth to a black child. His defense is recounted by Paré in *On Monsters and Marvels:* "Her husband and
she both having white skin . . . the woman was absolved upon
Hippocrates' persuasion that [her child] was [caused by] the por-
trait of a Moor, similar to the child, which was customarily attached to her bed."[16]

Other suggestions of perceived sexual deviance creep into these
stories, too. In *A Cabinet of Medical Curiosities*, Jan Bondeson
tells the story of a thirteenth-century noblewoman in Ursini who
gave birth to a child with the fur and paws of a bear. The defect
was blamed on a picture of a bear that hung in the woman's bedchamber. In the late fifteenth or early sixteenth century, Leon-
ardo da Vinci would famously echo this logic in his *Quaderni
d'anatomia:* "The things desired by the mother are often found
impressed on the child that which the mother carries at the time
of the desire." A mother shamed because of her sexual hunger.[17]

You are wives. You are mothers. You are defined by your relationship to others. You think for your baby now. You dress for
your baby now. You eat for your baby now. Anything you do for
yourself is selfish.

I have a friend who had one glass of wine a week during her pregnancy. Okay, I have a couple of friends who have done this. Each of them drank the wine to help them relax. And because it's fine and because it's safe and because, well, why do they even have to justify what they did?

I had wine when my first child was in her third trimester. I was experiencing back pain and my doctor told me to drink a little bit of wine and take a bath. I did it, but I kept it hidden.

Mothers who take antidepressants also find themselves pulled by these tensions. The effects on a developing fetus of antidepressants medically necessary for the well-being of the mother aren't fully known. So, mothers often receive conflicting advice. Many doctors warn a mother of the risks and then let her decide. During my first pregnancy, I took Zoloft, an antidepressant, and stayed on the drug throughout the pregnancy. During my second, I was off Zoloft, but found myself struggling. I wanted to go back on, but when I spoke with my doctor, I felt paralyzed by the fear of harming my child. The choice was mine, and I chose not to take the drug. I regret it often when I think back to that difficult pregnancy, endured while parenting a two-year-old, and everything that came after. My anger, irritation, lack of patience. Maybe it wouldn't have been better with Zoloft, but I wanted, just once, for my doctor to look at me and say, "You know there are risks to your child, but here are the risks to you if you don't take it."

Or maybe what I wanted was someone to look at me and say, "You are the expert on what you need. Take what you need. It's okay."

Eve's craving for forbidden food broke open the world. And from that bite came the curse of Eve—the pain of pregnancy. God, finding Eve hiding in shame in the garden curses her: "I will greatly multiply thy sorrow and thy conception: in sorrow thou shalt bring forth children."

The pain of motherhood, then, is a curse resulting from our indulgence as women, for the crime of eating. The crime of being so bold as to open your mouth and relieve your hunger, your craving. The curse of motherhood goes back to eating.

It's at this moment in mythology, the moment a woman ate exactly what she wanted when she wanted, when the agony of childbirth entered the world. Think of all those diets that exist to curb the food you eat. To control the passion and want and need growing inside you. We moralize about the foods women eat. Declaring some foods to be clean, good, and others, bad, sinful. This language of absolutism restricts women's appetites. It's no wonder that women in America by and large crave what is "bad"—salt, fat, sugar, fast food. The greasy delight of a hamburger, the warmth of a crisp fry. The cool, sweet rush of a cola. The sweet tang of ketchup.

I gave birth to my son in July. Right at the moment when I thought my body would burst. Everything was heavy and damp. The sweaty chafe of my thighs. The slick heat from between my breasts. Whenever I could, I would sneak away to buy a large Coke from the McDonald's drive-through. I'd drive to the park and sit in the car listening to top 40 radio, enjoying the delicious feel of no one touching me, the cold sweetness down my throat. No one asking when I was due. No one shouting, as a man at Home Depot had, "Should you even be walking?" To which I had snapped, "Should you?"

We hunger for what we've been forbidden.

As the inheritors of Eve's eternal punishment, we bear the burden of redeeming ourselves. A tract from 1830 opines of mothers: "She who was first in the transgression, must yet be the principal earthly instrument in the restoration. It is maternal influence, after all, which must be the great agent in the hands of God, in bringing back our guilty race to duty and happiness."[18] So we must always be making up for, through restraint, what the first woman did through excess.

And so our hunger is restricted, and our children become our way to access our hunger.

A friend tells me her doctor switched the office scale to kilograms so that American mothers couldn't easily do the math to figure out their weight. An offer of freedom to consume. To desire. To grow. That life inside you is an excuse to be fully alive and fully hungry in a way you never were before. And together with that child you are allowed to ache for food and drink and fullness in a way you never let yourself be before.

I wish this had been my experience. With my doctor, with the rest of the world. Perhaps it was because I so visibly gained weight. I had always—by virtue of genetics and an anxious proclivity to forget to eat—been thin. So, I went from a very thin woman to a fat one. Which is just to say, I gained weight. There ought to be no moral tinge to the word *fat*. Bodies are just bodies, perfect in their existence. Our experiences with them are varying. But as women in America we are lashed to them. Our self-worth and value are knotted up in how we present to the world. And so *fat* often does carry a moral judgment. Gaining weight is a sin in our society, which condemns weight as immoral, evidence of a personal failing.

As a thin woman, eating Cheetos was a joke. People smiled. They laughed when I spoke of it. As a fat woman, even pregnant, eating Cheetos wasn't a joke. I felt suddenly observed. My every mouthful watched.

"Are you sure that's what you want to eat?" a family member asked me when I ate chips while watching a Christmas movie. I was six months pregnant.

It's no wonder, then, that our appetites are fraught. It's no wonder our wombs are caught in this tangle of desire, hunger, and shame. In searching for answers, I found multiple scientific studies on how to help pregnant women suppress their appetites, how to encourage them to eat "healthier." The danger, the studies suggested, was the baby itself gaining weight.

Oster analyzed the research on maternal weight gain in relation to the size of the baby. Weight gained did somewhat correlate with the weight of the newborn. But there are risks to not gaining enough weight, too. "Both very large and very small babies face additional risks, although too small babies face greater risks. If anything, you should probably be more concerned about gaining too little weight than too much. . . . But, mostly, just chill out," Oster concludes.[19]

Eat, Oster's research suggests. Eat.

Jewish mythology tells us that before Eve, a woman named Lilith existed. She was Adam's first wife, cast out of the Garden because she demanded equality with man. Lilith personifies the female evil—the tempting serpent in the Garden, the reason men spill their seed (the biblical euphemism for masturbation, if you must know). She is a night hag, a monster, a demon, the mother of demons, the lover of Satan. She is a vampire, a succubus. Some stories claim the angels placed a curse on her that every day a hundred of her demon seed would die as a punishment for her evil nature. In revenge, she tries to kill the children of Eve. She is credited as the cause of stillborns. She is the patron demon of abortions.

Lilith hungers for and consumes children, while Eve must bear children because she hungered. In punishment, Eve is restrained. A good woman now. But Lilith is all appetite. Her hunger destroys children.

In *Sisters at Sinai: New Tales of Biblical Women*, a feminist rereading of women in the Bible, Jill Hammer retells the story of Lilith and Eve. Instead of rivals, they become partners. In

Hammer's version, Lilith lures Eve to the center of the Garden and tells Eve that she lives in the ocean, where she gives birth to children who are stolen by the angels. Lilith explains that her children are the souls of Eve's children and, in order for them to live, Eve must eat of the forbidden fruit. To illustrate her point, Lilith creates a fire that heats the forbidden fruit until it bursts "like seed pods" and thousands of tiny lights scatter into the night.

Lilith then says, "We are meant to scatter our sparks in the world. Without that task, we are not alive. And so you must begin death, and hope, and children. You must bear bodies for the souls that are waiting."[20]

Hunger, then, in this retelling, does not curse humanity but rather gives us life. Eve's eating seizes the labor of creation from the hands of a patriarchal God and puts it inside the womb. She bears children who unite with the souls that Lilith creates. Eating is the process through which soul and flesh are united.

Yet, we cannot allow women to eat. Because what then? What if we stop suppressing their appetites? What if we allow them to consume fully and without reproach? Well, maybe they would consume the world or maybe they would create it.

I want us to write a new myth about hunger. I want a new story.

It might seem a foolish, useless act to try to tell these stories again. We like to think we are a modern society and don't base our rules and restrictions on religious myths. And yet, why are our taboos about women so varying, so tied to culture? Why is a woman eating what she wants such a radical act? Why is it especially radical when that woman has a life in her? Maybe retelling a myth could be a starting point for reimagining how we understand our science and all of its biases.

So, I ask for new stories. I want us to tell stories about how Eve is allowed to eat. How her desire for that fruit is not a curse but a gift. How her hunger is her wholeness. How her consumption and her fullness are part of her power, not its destruction. How the end of Eden is the beginning of Eve. I want a story in which food is not the danger but the salvation. I want a story in which the God character is sinister and the snake is freedom. I want a story in which Eve slurping the juices of that fruit is an act of protest and fulfillment. And I want us not just to tell these stories but also to braid them into our cultural mythology.

Each time I was pregnant, I wanted to eat everything. I wanted to open my mouth and let everything flow in. My first pregnancy, I resisted. Despite my restraint, I still gained over fifty pounds. And with each appointment, my doctor's mouth would stretch into a thin line as she fussed over the reasons for my weight gain. By the end of my pregnancy, I had acid reflux and felt so uncomfortable I ate fruit and water. It didn't help. I still gained weight.

But the time I was pregnant with my son, I stopped caring. My body seemed to want to expand and contract and who was I to stop it? I ate the sandwiches almost nightly for six months. I gained over fifty pounds, but I didn't worry. This time I let myself eat, like I never had before. I let my body dictate its relationship with the physical world. I saw myself expand, saw my skin stretch. I'd often dream that people came to me and offered me plates of food, their pets, their aging loved ones, and I'd gently draw them all into my mouth. The process of eating the world felt like an outpouring of love. If I could draw everything into me, everything would be safe.

Because within me was a vast and unknowable world, dark and protective. So, I consumed and fed that space in me and I watched myself grow. I did not feed the baby. I fed myself. Because we were one at that moment, part of an intricate and mysterious process.

I made the sandwich again recently. I constructed it as faithfully as possible, given that it was February and no good tomatoes were to be found. Still, I layered seeded rye, mayo, tomatoes sprinkled with salt, a smear of mustard, iceberg lettuce, thick deli turkey, kosher dill pickles. I cut it in half.

I was alone. My kids were with their father for the night. (We have joint custody.) I am a different sort of mother than I was when I had my first child. I'm a different sort of human. I am angrier. I'm also leaner. I ran a lot during my divorce and stopped cooking. I finally did lose that baby weight. People would ask me how I did it, and I'd say, "I let myself be angry. I got divorced." They'd laugh. But it wasn't a joke. Those rage-propelled workouts changed my body.

I like my body more now. Not because of its weight, but because of its strength. I once carried an entire bookcase from my car to my living room, alone. With strength comes freedom. And I want to be free. I want to be a mother, a body, that pushes to exist without constraint, an impossible goal. How can you be fully free of everything? Every cultural pull, every patriarchal impulse?

If I got pregnant now, would I have more than one secret glass of wine during the third trimester? Would I have sushi? Would I eat?

I want to say yes. I want to say I would open my mouth and let the world fall in. But I don't know. Eating, truly eating—without worry, without the constant tangle of culture and science and mythology—it's something I cannot comprehend.

This sandwich—was it just a craving? Some sort of weird chemical thing that only happened during pregnancy? Maybe I had just been tricked into being hungry by the changes in my body. Maybe it was a salt craving. Maybe it was the momentary chemical imbalance of the pregnancy.

I ate the sandwich. And it was good.

Desire

When she was pregnant, Michelle Wilkins had her picture taken in a Colorado meadow. It's late fall, and Wilkins stands in a field of golden prairie grass. The photos show her glowing, draped in a thick cream-colored sweater and adorned with a crown of russet flowers and dark green leaves. In one image she cradles her stomach, the orbs of her white cheeks wide with happiness. Her eyes are cast down, a rope of pearls dripping from her neck. Her baby's name was Aurora.[1]

In March 2015, two months before her due date, and just a couple of months after those pictures were taken, Wilkins went to the home of Dynel Lane in Longmont, Colorado, to pick up some maternity clothes Lane had advertised in a Craigslist ad. The two women got along immediately, talking and laughing about children and pregnancy. Lane was older than Wilkins and had two teenage daughters and a son, who thirteen years earlier had died when he was nineteen months old in an accidental drowning. She was pregnant too. Her tubes had been tied, but there she was, pregnant. It was a miracle of sorts.

Lane led Wilkins to the basement, where the clothes were, and then the mood changed. Wilkins remembers Lane acting different, suddenly nervous, and then attacking her. Lane smashed a lava lamp over Wilkins's head and began to choke her, pressing her hand on Wilkins's throat. She stabbed her, too, cutting her open from hip to hip with kitchen knives, tearing out baby Aurora. Wilkins, who survived the attack, said she could feel her intestines outside of her body.[2]

Lane had taken pregnancy pictures too. These smiling mirror selfies predate the attack by just a few weeks and show Lane, with smooth brown hair, cradling the rising mound of her stomach, which is pressing out against her brown peasant-style top. She had named the child James.

Lane put Aurora's small body in the bathtub. Then she cleaned up from the attack. Doing laundry, washing up the blood. Wilkins was in the basement, left for dead. Lane took the baby to the hospital, saying it was hers, saying the baby was stillborn. Meanwhile, Wilkins managed to call 911 and was rushed from the scene of the crime to the hospital.

Later examinations showed Lane hadn't been pregnant. Not then, anyway. But friends and family would say she was obsessed with pregnancy to an unhealthy degree. During the trial, her lawyer argued that the grief of loss and the desire to become a mother had driven Lane to her crime.[3]

In 2016, Lane was convicted of attempted murder and unlawful termination of a pregnancy and sentenced to a hundred years in prison.

Fetal abduction is a rare but disproportionately American crime. Since 1974, at least twenty-two women have attempted to cut open the uterus of another woman and steal the child from within. Reported cases in other countries are rare.

In an interview with the *Chicago Tribune*, Theresa Porter, a psychologist who studies fetal abductions, noted that the women are motivated by the special treatment they receive when they claim they're pregnant: "You don't have to do some things like housework, maybe, and you do get some other things like a foot rub or a back rub. It comes down to attention. You're the center of attention. Everyone's doing things for you. And this seemed to be a big issue for a lot of these women." Women who lie about pregnancy, Porter argues, are not simply lying, they are creating a fictional world in which they and their bodies are the center. They believe this story, but it's a fairy tale with a time limit of nine months.[4]

For so many women, pregnancy is an honor—the canonization of a certain type of femininity. Often, it's the only time that society celebrates a woman, besides her wedding. There are baby showers. Pregnancy photos. Gifts. Special food. Special attention. People on the subway give up their seat for you. Men hold open doors. When I was six months pregnant with my daughter, I went on a trip to New York to visit the offices of the love and relationships website I was working for at the time. Everyone was so kind. Cabs pulled over for me. People moved out of my way. I joked with my boss that I could murder someone in Central Park and get away with it simply by pointing to my belly and shrugging.

The next time I was in New York, a year later and very unpregnant, I got shoved into the street. Pregnant, I had been special. Unpregnant, I was just another annoying white tourist who didn't know how to navigate the subway.

Pregnancy is power. Our culture bestows esteem and honor upon women who conceive and carry children. Fawning over and fetishizing the rising tide of our bellies.

"Pregnancy is the first time in life I felt really important," my neighbor Stephanie confesses. Stephanie is the mother of four children. She was an Evangelical Christian, and she clung to that faith, which provided reassurance and structure to her life. But with each birth, she began to question the demands from her church that she submit to the authority of her husband and white male church leaders.

"When I saw what my body could do, what I could do," she told me one day as we watched our children play together at the park, "I just woke up. I realized I knew what I needed more than any of those men."

Her whole life growing up in Mississippi, Stephanie had been told that her body was a problem. She had to cover it up. Be pure. Act right. Now, a mother, her body had purpose, and through that purpose she found her voice. She began to ask for what she needed. Her youngest child was born with a midwife, who was attentive to Stephanie and who followed her birth plan, something none of Stephanie's obstetricians had done. Stephanie isn't the first, nor is she the last, to find power in pregnancy.

My own mother had eight children, of which I am the second oldest. Eight children in sixteen years meant that she was pregnant through much of the eighties and nineties. My mother's sentiments echo Stephanie's: with each pregnancy and each birth, she found a sense of power and purpose. She allowed herself to speak over the demands of a hospital system that was often unsympathetic to her wants and desires. By the time my brother Caleb, number six, came along in 1993, my mother gave birth in a midwife center in Dallas. There, she says, she finally had a birth experience that left her feeling cared for and listened to.

Growing a baby, pregnant women feel empowered to ask for things they'd never dared, or even considered, asking for before. Amy Richardson, cofounder of Third Wave Feminism, notes that pregnancy is one of the first times many women feel entitled to ask for things like space and rest. And it's one of the few times that our society allows women to take those things for themselves. We insist on it. *Sit in this seat. Put your feet up. Take care of yourself.*

But is it the woman or the baby that we are truly caring for? After all, once the baby is successfully delivered, separated from mother, the care and the urgency we have for the mother body suddenly vanish, subsumed by care and urgency for the infant.

In 2017, Beyoncé performed at the Grammy's pregnant and draped in gold, a gold headband that crowned her head like the sun's rays. She was a goddess, her body brilliant and powerful, containing not just one child, but twins. I watched the performance with tears in my eyes. It felt like a vision of power of all a woman could be.

The next morning, at the gym a woman grumpily complained that she hated the performance. "You'd think Beyoncé invented being pregnant," she said.

It was a petty comment, oblivious to the context. Black mothers are more likely to die from childbirth than are white mothers, are more likely to be questioned or condescended to by doctors. Beyoncé was making a statement of competence and autonomy in a world that would take them from her. From the gold flowing gown to the starburst headband, Beyoncé's iconography of power was resonant because it tapped into the abiding mythology of mother as goddess. Early carvings of deities show women with exaggerated breasts, stomachs, and vulvas. Mother goddesses of fertility and life. In the Hindu religion, the mother goddess is Durga, one aspect of the Brahma; she is before life, and after life; she is the conduit of life.

But Beyoncé's performance of goddess is still a performance. In later interviews, she spoke candidly about her pregnancy and her body and the struggle. It was anything but a golden spectacle. But that moment of seizing power had meaning because it's a power not often given to black mothers in America.

Birth is power. It's the only reliable way humans can make life (for now). To have a womb is to control the means of human production. Our blood, our bodies, our capability for giving life, which Christ named the source of a woman's power.

The movie *Children of Men*, based on the novel by P. D. James, imagines a world where decades of infertility have left human society desperate and dying. Clive Owen plays a civil servant who must protect a young refugee named Kee, the first woman to become pregnant in decades, so she can make it to a scientific community dedicated to solving the fertility crisis and, somehow, save humanity. There is a moment in the movie when the two have to make their way through a battle between the refugees and the soldiers. When the people see Kee's belly, they stop and stare, their awe for the life in her quelling their fear and rage.

I felt like that when I was pregnant. Walking into a room with a stomach swollen with life is a powerful thing. People stop and stare. Strangers smile. You're treated with a kind of reverence.

Pregnancy feels like power because it is. But it is a tenuous power.

It's tenuous because of the anxieties that arise from that power. The pregnant body is a palimpsest for our cultural anxieties. There, writ large over the belly of a mother, are all of our fears and anxieties and hopes and virtues.

The power of pregnant women is analogous to the power we give to veterans. In many grocery stores throughout the country, the best parking spaces are reserved for "Veterans" and "Expecting Mothers." Veterans and people with small children are allowed to board first on airplanes. But like the honor we give veterans, it's a shallow regard. One that is predicated on the sacrifice of one's body for one's country. Veterans can get discounts at stores and restaurants, but they still struggle to access adequate healthcare. And we discard that body once that body has done its duty. Women who are no longer pregnant are mothers, necessary but cumbersome to society. And we sublimate their power into their role. They are now no longer a woman, but a mother, important primarily for the role they play in someone else's life.

One of my least favorite aspects of motherhood is being introduced as the mother of my child. I understand the functional use of this designation, and yet. The role of mama, mommy, mother of my child strips me of my other functions and powers. Once I walk into the room as a mother, I am not a writer. I am not the woman who can run a mile in less than six minutes. I am not a complete person. I am merely a conduit for another person, another life. Therein lies my significance. I am proud of my children. I often tell them they are the best stories I've ever written. But the truth is, they are their own people—part of my story, but fully their own, separate from me. Nothing has heightened this realization more than divorce.

When my children were four and six, their father and I separated. Before, I had been the primary parent. Organizing their lives. Volunteering at school. Waking up with them in the morning, putting them to bed at night. I was their everything: their cook, their cleaner, their party planner, their butt wiper. Then, one day, in November 2017, that changed. Suddenly, I had whole days without them. And they had days, important moments and experiences, that I was not present for.

So, I, who had been first and foremost a mother, had to become a mother in absentia. A mother who is without. And that, too, became a role. Only this role had no power; this role conferred shame.

I was the divorced mom out drinking on a weeknight with a man. The divorced mom working feverishly into the weekend. Every choice was tainted with the emptiness of my absence from my role. It all felt a little desperate. As if I was supposed to only engage in activities that would pull me back into that role of full-time mother.

"Who is watching the children?" and "Who is with the children?" were the constant refrains of men and women who saw me out on dates with friends or romantic partners. They're familiar to many mothers who have dared to do something, anything, without the constant presence of their children. The role of a mother whose children are outside of her womb is less about her and more about them.

As my marriage was falling apart, a new show called *The Handmaid's Tale* was released. Based on Margaret Atwood's novel by the same name, the show premiered in April 2017, right after Donald Trump became president and the push to overturn *Roe v. Wade* became more than just a campaign promise and quickly became a cultural touchpoint. I couldn't watch it. I tried. But at the time, grappling with my Evangelical past and my religious spouse, the show didn't present a vision of dystopia for me but the actual reality I was living in.

The narrative Atwood presents explores the complex power and potential of pregnancy. Set in a theocracy called Gilead, where pollution has made fertility rare, women have been captured and forced to play one of three roles: homemaker, servant, or Handmaid—the surrogates for wealthy and powerful couples. Both bound because of their ability to conceive and made powerful by it, the Handmaids occupy a dangerous political space. As such, they are tightly controlled, brainwashed during their training. But they're also given certain freedoms and rewards for doing their duties. The narrator, Offred, muses, "A rat in a maze is free to go anywhere, as long as it stays inside the maze."

The power of pregnancy in the United States is like the power of a Handmaid in Gilead, power subdued and power restrained. When I was seventeen years old, a pastor at Bible camp explained to me and a group of other girls that our power was like that of a horse: better when broken in and restrained. He might as well have said the power of a rat, inside of a cage.

Like Handmaids, caged rats, and trained horses, pregnant women are dismissed once their duty is done. In the worst cases, they are disposed of. During Argentina's "Dirty War," the government imprisoned pregnant women and forced them to deliver. The children were then given to wealthy citizens who supported the regime. The women, the biological mothers, were murdered.[5]

During my first pregnancy, I was addicted to the message boards on Bump.com. I'd log in every morning after I woke up and scroll through story after story of women asking sometimes-silly questions ("Can the baby see my husband's penis when we have sex?") as well as more serious ones ("I'm bleeding, should I go to the hospital?"). The boards were organized by due date. I joined the one for women due to give birth in March 2011. I got to know the other women—by their handles, by their concerns. One woman's pregnancy seemed to be a constant spiral of pain and fear. Her boyfriend wasn't supportive. She was often bleeding. She'd had miscarriages before. Every post was mired in tragedy, in concern, all centered on her womb.

Then, one morning, when we were about five months pregnant, another woman posted a thread accusing this woman of being a fake. She'd done some investigating and learned this woman had faked pregnancies before. Her posts were all a play for power. With her body's potential, she'd created a world where she was the center of a daily drama.

I never saw the pregnancy faker on the boards again. Maybe she left, or maybe she changed her screen name. Maybe she joined another board, created another world, where she was significant, where she had control, where she mattered.

Habek Dubravko, of the Department of Obstetrics and Gyne-
cology at the School of Medicine Sveti Duh General Hospital in
Croatia, published a study of pseudocyesis, or false pregnancy, in
2010. In the article, she describes a fifty-nine-year-old woman
who was rushed to the hospital screaming she was going to "give
birth to little Jesus." She was a single woman, a devout Catholic
who lived with her family. She insisted she was pregnant and she
looked it, too. "Her breasts were enlarged and tumescent wide
gait due to the large, prominent abdomen." Her mind had, in a
way, impregnated her body.[6]

Though false pregnancy is rare, it has been seen in women
throughout history. Hippocrates noted twelve such cases. There
is a persistent historical rumor that Mary I, Queen of England,
also known as Mary Tudor, suffered from pseudocyesis. Some
historians—men, probably—surmise that her infamous bloody
rages were spurned by her realizations that she was not, in fact,
pregnant.

Reductive historical analysis aside, psychologists believe that
fake pregnancies are motivated by an overwhelming desire for
children. I wonder, though, if sometimes it's not an overwhelming desire for children, but for pregnancy, and the power and
agency it affords women.

The power of pregnancy is not accessible to all women, or
even all pregnant people. Our culture punishes people who are
trans, nonbinary, or butch for transgressing gender norms. The
power of femininity is a power more easily given to those who
read as middle- and upper-class straight white women. But even
for those women, femininity is a trap. Some women, of course,
choose not to be pregnant—a power in its own right. But others,
who want to conceive and can't, describe feeling powerless.

The problem with centering the womb as the woman's path
to goddess-hood is that it completely devalues a woman's other

achievements and contributions to the world. In 2013, when rocket scientist Yvonne Brill died, her obituary in the *New York Times* focused on her role as wife and mother and maker of a really good beef stroganoff. The internet responded in its usually calm and measured way. Just kidding—there was a huge outcry, on Twitter and elsewhere, prompting a discussion of how we see and venerate women. The *Times* changed the obituary to de-emphasize her stroganoff relative to her contributions to science. Writing in the *Times*, public editor Margaret Sullivan noted that the author of the obituary had set up the description of Brill's domestic life as a bait and switch so that the "aha" moment of her scientific discoveries in the second paragraph would read as surprising. The author, a man, commented that he thought the outcry was "unwarranted."[7]

Of course he did. Never would it occur to him to ask whether framing a man as a father and incredible cooker of Hamburger Helper would lead to an "aha" moment when he's also named as a brilliant novelist. It's a tired argument, but one we clearly have to keep making. Men are allowed to be more than fathers. Whereas women, if we are mothers, that is all we are allowed to be.

And if we are not mothers, if we choose to do other things, our lives always raise the unanswered question posed by the existence of our wombs.

A friend of mine, another mother, who I was close with before my divorce, when my life was centered on home and children, came to the housewarming for the home I bought as a single woman and writer. When I asked her about her life, about all the things that had happened in the three years since we'd spent time with one another, she sighed. "You know how it is," she said. "At some point, your life is just all about kids."

I knew she was right in so many ways. Not only the house we stood in but also many of my other life choices were all about my children. But my friend was also wrong. It wasn't just about the kids. There was more and I was more. The truth of my life was that I could create life and love the humans I made and still have a world bigger than them. A world that contained me as more than them.

It can be freeing to find power in your womb. But if that is the extent of the power we allow women, it's not really power at all. We set up the rest of our lives and accomplishments to be a grand "aha" moment, an afterthought compared to our children and beef stroganoff. What I am doing here, this is not an "aha" moment. My children, my womb, the nachos I make every week— those are not the setup for the irony that I've achieved something more, that my life is more.

In a *New York Times Magazine* dual profile of the artists Celia Paul and Cecily Brown, Rachel Cusk takes issue with the narrative that Brown creates about her work, when she remarks that if she never achieves all she can be as a professional, it's because she chose to be a mother. Cusk contradicts her, writing, "Motherhood is an inextricable aspect of female being; it is one thing to choose not to have a child at all, but if you can do both, be both, then surely the possibility of formulating a grander female vision and voice becomes graspable."[8]

Cusk is trying to push back against the narrative that a woman is less as an artist because she's a mother. But in doing so, she falls into the trap of the mother as goddess and possessor of power. A grander female voice is not only within the grasp of those who perform the role of mother. I have no more insight, no more voice or vision, just because I used my uterus twice to make humans.

And even now, to write this feels like I am transgressing. I feel like I have to assure you that of course I love my children, I would die for them. But they are not my everything. They are not all I have. They are not all I am. And I am not all I am because of them. They are still woven into me, but it's part of a more complex thread of life and relationships.

The fallacy of this line of thinking is also evident from the side of those who want to be mothers but who cannot find their way into that role. The power of the womb also leads to powerlessness when a womb cannot be used. Alison, a friend of mine, struggled with fertility for almost a decade, going through three rounds of in vitro fertilization treatments. On our coffee dates, she'd complain to me about friends and well-meaning acquaintances who would tell her just to "relax" and stop wanting babies so much. Person after person would tell her about their friend or relative who couldn't have a baby, and then the moment they stopped trying, boom! They had one. Just like that. For Alison, these stories made her feel ashamed. As if she had transgressed in her desire. As if it was the wanting of a child that deemed her unworthy. There was also a sense of powerlessness. As if everything in her life, all her accomplishments, all her relationships, all her lived victories and disappointments never mattered, only this one thing, this act of conception.

Later, when I divorced and began dating again, I lamented that no suitable dates were to be found, and people doled out similar advice to me: *You can't want it too much. You have to just live your life, and then, boom, it'll happen.* Just like that. Marriage and children are milestones, desired, valued, and celebrated in almost every aspect of our culture, and yet we are demeaned for seeking them. For striving for them. As if we had trespassed merely by wanting.

For much of history, before we understood the biology (and sometimes even now), the inability to conceive a child was viewed as a curse. God's disfavor on a woman for her sins or her husband's. The Hebrew Bible includes story after story of women crying out to the Lord to open their wombs so that they could bear a child. One example is the story of Hannah, which takes place in 1 Samuel. Hannah is the first wife of a man named El-kanah. Because Hannah was childless, Elkanah took a second wife, Peninnah. The childless woman and the mother are mir-ror roles in the Hebrew Bible to the stories of Rachel and Leah, Sarah and Hagar. Through these parallels we see the relative power of these roles in stark contrast: those with children have the power and status; those without must turn to the Lord.

Mocked by Peninnah, Hannah goes to the temple to pray. Offering her child to the Lord if he would only bless her with a child. She is so blessed. The Lord remembers her and opens her womb, and she bears the prophet Samuel, who, after he is weaned, she gives to the priest Eli. Samuel's birth bestows upon Hannah the recognition and status she so desperately desires, even more than she desires the child himself.

Hannah is the patron saint of women struggling with fertility, seen as selfless and loving. This is a story many people recited to Alison as an example of the selflessness of motherhood and the power of motherhood. One she quickly grew to hate during her rounds of IVF. But in Hannah I see a woman reduced. A woman for whom pregnancy is the means to an end. And who can blame her? In a world where her significance lay in the use of her uterus, where moral virtue and cultural power and love all depended on her ability to produce a child, of course that son was a means to an end.

Recent biblical scholars have questioned the universality of the desire for children in the Bible, arguing, in the words of Judith Butler, that "the category of women is normative and exclusion-ary . . . [and] the insistence upon the coherence and unity of the category of women has effectively refused the multiplicity of cul-tural, social, and political intersections in which the concrete way of 'women' are constructed."[9]

In other words, we presume Hannah wanted children and her desire was pure and her actions were selfless. There is no room, in the way this story is taught in many churches, to question whether it was in fact an act of cruelty to have a child, then dump him off at a temple to be raised by a cranky priest.

Hannah's story as presented is, in many ways, a reductive reading of a cultural myth, which is far more complex and nuanced than I am giving it credit for. Like so many women, Hannah's story has been flattened and reduced through the cultural engine that spits out our archetypes and holds them up for us to follow. But it is also the myth that was handed down to me as a child— one I heard in churches in Texas, Iowa, and South Dakota, the homes of my youth.

Biblical scholar Esther Fuchs writes that although it is tempting to see the story of Hannah as a story of power, it isn't. Motherhood for Hannah serves only to validate her role in a patriarchal society. "The literary constellation of male characters surrounding and determining the fate of the potential mother dramatizes the idea that woman's reproductive potential should be and can be controlled only by men."[10]

In that analysis, Fuchs encapsulates the entire problem. Motherhood is seen as powerful only when inside the confines of patriarchal norms. Motherhood on other terms—single motherhood, trans motherhood, queer motherhood, black or brown motherhood, non-motherhood—is transgressive.

The lessons of Hannah as they are taught exemplify the cultural narratives by which we uphold the value and power of pregnancy. "When are you having children?" "Do you want children?" "You should have children." These are the relentless slings and arrows our culture lobs at couples once they seem relatively happy and settled—or, increasingly, at single women of a certain age and stable income. As if children are all a woman could ever or should ever want. The message being that our fulfillment lies in our reproductive capabilities. In Sigrid Nunez's essay "The Most Important Thing," she writes, "That there could be something in the world that a woman could want more than children has been viewed as unacceptable. Things may be marginally different now, but, even if there is something she wants more than children, that is no reason for a woman to remain childless. Any normal woman, it is understood, wants—and should want—both."[11]

Women, pregnant or not, are often told what to want and why they should want it. Told to stay within the designated boundaries of what is deemed acceptable. Like rats wandering a maze, women have to stay within the confines of a complex system that asks us to twist in and out, looping back on ourselves and our desires.

For women, pregnancy is offered as the promise of fulfillment. And yet, to have a child, to raise one, comes with great loss of personal time, freedom, bodily autonomy, and financial resources. That loss can serve as cultural currency—fetishized as the martyrdom of motherhood. The status is not nothing. But it's the empty status of a "Veterans Only" parking spot. As mothers, we're told our loss is supposed to be our fulfillment. It's a twisted cultural logic, echoed by the voice of Aunt Lydia in *The Handmaid's Tale*, who undertakes her job to keep the Handmaids in line with violent zeal: "There is more than one kind of freedom . . . freedom to and freedom from. In the days of anarchy, it was freedom to. Now you are being given freedom from. Don't underrate it."[12]

In the two years following my divorce, I wanted a child so deeply and profoundly, it felt like a menstrual ache. It felt like a clenched fist inside of me. I'd rub my hips and lie on heating pads. Often, while falling asleep at night, I'd fantasize about my pregnancy, imagining midwife appointments, my bump distending in long flowing gowns. I imagined scenarios, parties, playdates, when people would ask me who the father of my unborn child was, and I'd smile and say, "Feminism." A joke that would also not be a joke. I felt this desire so deeply that I often asked other divorced women if they felt the same way.

"No, are you crazy?" was the almost universal response.

And then, one day, holding my friend's deliciously chubby circle of a baby in a Mexican restaurant, the desire disappeared. It could have been the muscle memory of the exhaustion, the pain, the fear, the loss of time and freedom. The full weight of the reality of what pregnancy actually meant. Or maybe it was because I'd had time to grieve the loss of my marriage. And once that grief had been dealt with, I no longer felt the desire for a child. Or maybe, too, I had wanted a child because I felt like I wanted to reclaim my body and its power. I had felt my loss of social status as a married woman. Perhaps wanting a child was a way of trying to reclaim a more elevated social status? And in holding that beautiful child, spending time with my friend, I remembered that I had other ways of understanding my power, outside of the context of my womb.

Sanity

It's not hard to gaslight a pregnant person. Tell them they're on their period. Tell them it's hormones. Tell them the baby is making them act different. They're not themselves. They're not in their right mind.

It's not hard because it's not wrong—not exactly. Having a baby changes a person. Mothers I know have had their hair change. Or their eyesight. Their feet have grown. They've eaten foods they never would have eaten before. The smell of their beloved partner now fills them with rage and nausea.

There are other changes, too. The small shifts in memory, in focus, in priorities. And the cataclysmic changes in body, space, time. During both of my pregnancies, my breasts went from an A cup to an E cup. It was a seismic shift that completely changed how I dressed, stood, walked, and navigated the world. A woman with nursing boobs walks through the world in a fundamentally different way from how a woman who doesn't even need to wear a bra does.

Scientists seem to universally conclude that pregnancy and birth alter a woman in ways that we still don't fully understand.

Studies in rats show that memory and the ability to learn increase after pregnancy.[1] Our brain structure changes.[2] When the cells of the baby enter our body, in a process that scientists refer to as microchimerism, we become part ourselves, part other. How all this affects us is still largely a mystery.

So, it's not hard to gaslight a pregnant woman. It's not hard to tell her that she's changed, that something isn't right with her, that she isn't right. After all, look at her body. Look at the way it shifts and changes. Look at how it oozes blood and hormones. Her hair, once curly and now straight. Once straight, but now curly. Parts of her brain fundamentally shifted. Her cells permanently changed.

Who can even recognize her?

The movie *Rosemary's Baby* is a story about fear, betrayal, and a good old-fashioned evil cult. The movie is shot from the point of view of Rosemary, played by Mia Farrow, a young woman who is happily married and moves with her husband into a new apartment with some weird neighbors. The night she conceives, Rosemary is drugged with chocolate mousse and has visions of being raped by a demon. Her husband tells her he had sex with her while she was unconscious (which is also called rape). She's upset and vulnerable and confused. Rosemary loses weight, craves raw chicken and liver, drinks a weird health drink mixed by one of her weird new neighbors. She begins to suspect the building is full of Satanists who are part of a coven. She tries to tell her doctor, who dismisses her fears and calls her hysterical. Roman Polanski, who directed the film, and who was also credibly accused of rape, leaves little room for ambiguity about what is happening to Rosemary. It's clear the director is not questioning her sanity—the baby is born the child of the Devil himself.

When Mia Farrow took the role, it made her husband, Frank Sinatra, so mad he divorced her. It's not that he hated the movie; he hated her working.

The film has been interpreted as a feminist horror story. A cautionary tale of a woman's body being completely consumed by the evil intentions and powers of others. For me, it has always felt more like a documentary, an encapsulation of pregnancy— disorienting, bizarre, sinister, with cravings that make just as much sense as raw chicken, dismissive doctors, and condescendingly cloying neighbors. The horror comes less from haunting "what ifs" than from the eerie parallels to pregnancy.

It wasn't hard to gaslight me. I went on Zoloft a month before I found out I was pregnant with my daughter. My parents had split up and were in the throes of a midlife crisis, which they handled by calling their children and complaining about each other. I had just graduated from my master's program. We'd decided to have a baby. I began feeling like I was having heart attacks. I cried over the fact that I had failed to pick up a dress from the dry cleaner's before it closed. My friend, who had just gone through postpartum depression, told me to see a doctor. The doctor put me on Zoloft and gave me Xanax for my heart attacks, which were actually panic attacks. She said sometimes life ruins us a bit, but I would be fine.

Five years and one more kid later, I was off the meds, but my husband was telling me I should go back on. That I was crazy. "Your hormones changed you," he said. "You need medication for your emotions."

And: "I don't recognize you. Maybe it's your thyroid?"

I googled thyroid problems. I googled depression and bipolar disorder. Was I okay? Was I losing my mind? Was I losing myself?

When women do struggle with genuine issues, such as bipolar disorder and hyperthyroidism, they are often overlooked and misdiagnosed. They're told it's their hormones, that they're fine. They have to insist on treatment. But here I was, insisting I was fine and being told I needed treatment. I spoke to doctors and therapists, who told me I was fine. At home I felt like I was going crazy. Household items were going missing. Everything I did was wrong.

It's not hard to gaslight a vulnerable person.

In Emily Brontë's *Wuthering Heights*, Catherine Linton goes insane over the course of her pregnancy. The novel follows the story of Catherine and Heathcliff, who was adopted into her family and raised as her sibling until he was relegated to an adult life as a servant. He runs away when Catherine marries Edgar Linton. When Heathcliff returns, educated and rich, Catherine is pregnant. Her husband demands that she stop seeing Heathcliff. "It is impossible for you to be my friend and his at the same time," Linton insists. Catherine, torn between the two men, answers that she "requires to be let alone." She dashes her head against the sofa. Alternating between rage and despair, she lays out as if she is dead, but only for a moment, before she sits up, "her hair flying over her shoulders, her eyes flashing, the muscles of her neck and arms standing out preternaturally."[3]

She locks herself in her room. When she emerges she has lost herself. She looks in a mirror and is incapable of recognizing her own face.

As her pregnancy progresses, so does her madness. At one point, Catherine rips a pillow to pieces, scattering the feathers, as Ophelia once scattered flowers in *Hamlet*.

As she flings the feathers, she calls out their names. "That's a turkey's . . . and this is a wild duck's; and this is a pigeon's. . . . And here's a moor-cock's."[4]

Whereas Ophelia's madness was tied to her deflowering, Catherine's insanity is tied to her pregnancy and her marriage. She is no longer the "wild, hatless little savage" she was with Heathcliff in her childhood. She is a wife and a mother and, as such, she must become docile. But the cost of her docility is her soul.

By the time she gives birth, she is an empty shell of her former self.

Wuthering Heights was Emily Brontë's only novel. A recluse who lived a short and tragic life, Emily knew too well the brutalities of flesh. As a child, she had watched her own mother die of ovarian cancer—her agony prolonged over seven months. She was trained in the brutal religion of English schools, which considered the corporeal body sin incarnate. Of course, this context extends beyond Brontë's era. That her character would go mad under the burden of domestic expectations makes just as much sense now as it did then.

The insanity of pregnancy appears in medical texts as a disease in the 1820s and 1830s. In *A Cultural History of Pregnancy*, Clare Hanson argues that the diagnosis of insanity of pregnancy was a cultural creation, a term that encompassed the anxieties of a condition that could kill a woman, trap her into domestic servitude, or, depending on her circumstances, ruin her moral character. Pregnancy could kill a woman. And even if she didn't die, her child likely would.[5]

Given those circumstances, it's not shocking that doctors noticed that women would become despondent and depressed while pregnant. They spun out the diagnosis as a melancholia, a temporary insanity, easily solved by birth—by the division of mother and child.

Creating a diagnosis for women's emotional state made it pathological, enabling doctors to control women, to put them away. I am sure these men thought they were doing right by the women. After all, *look at that woman, look at how irrational and unlike herself she is*. And they weren't entirely wrong, of course—that's what makes this so complicated, so hard to address.

Postpartum depression is a real condition, one that affects one in seven American mothers. Perinatal depression, or depression during pregnancy, is also a real and devastating condition. But we don't have good data on how many women experience perinatal depression. Studies have found that it is often overlooked and misdiagnosed, and that even when women are diagnosed, they don't usually receive treatment.[6] Perinatal depression is most prevalent among low-income women and women of color.[7] The reason women don't get help? Inaccessible healthcare, lack of healthcare, lack of community support, fear. There is also the cultural expectation that they be goddess warrior, pregnant power mamas.

John B. Tuke, in his 1867 paper "Cases Illustrative of the Insanity of Pregnancy, Puerperal Mania, and Insanity of Lactation," tells story after story of young mothers driven mad by their pregnancies. In one, a twenty-six-year-old woman identified as J. M. B. is relatively happy and healthy until her fifth pregnancy, during which she becomes melancholic and depressed, and then begins stealing. Tuke saw a direct line between the growth of her baby and the decline of her mind and morals. J. M. B. made a recovery after giving birth, but during her sixth pregnancy, she permanently lost herself. She was sent to a mental hospital after the birth, and Tuke writes, "No improvement in her mental condition. A more complete moral perversion could not exist in any one. She lies, steals, tells the nastiest stories without a blush, has not a grain of gratitude in her composition, invents the most dangerous stories against those who have been kindest to her, and seems, in fact, to be an incarnation of evil."[8]

This is Tuke's view of J. M. B.: a woman with moral perversion. A woman whose weak mind was driven insane by her pregnancies.

At the time of Tuke's writing, mothers were encouraged to control themselves. Don't think too hard. Don't read. Don't overexcite yourself with fun. No loud conversations. No thinking about anything beyond domestic labor. A woman who could not control herself, after all, was not fit to be a mother. John Abbott wrote in his 1835 pregnancy guide, "Can a mother expect to govern her child, when she cannot govern herself?"[9] The answer was to subdue the fever of their minds. Avoid novels. Stimulating activity. She was to keep a tight rein on the abundance of her body.

As science advanced, control remained the goal. Because women apparently couldn't be trusted to make good choices on their own, physicians took over the task of keeping them in line. The advice was still—as always—control yourself, woman.

The mysterious changes. The waxing moon of her womb. The fluid that escapes, unbidden. The desires, the cravings. All of these things were to be contained. After all, a good mother is a woman who keeps her legs closed and mind docile.

The fitness of our minds has always been tied to the extremes of our wombs. Although the insanity of pregnancy is a relatively modern diagnosis, Plato believed that a womb, especially one not otherwise occupied by babies, could wander throughout the body and cause any number of health problems, specifically hysteria. *Hysteria* was a catch-all for mood swings and undefined psychological problems. Through much of medical history the womb was defined as the source of this hysteria, this womanly madness. The seventeenth-century doctor William Harvey described the uterus as "insatiable, ferocious, animal-like," comparing "hysterical women" to "bitches in heat."[10]

After the seventeenth century, doctors learned that wombs stay in place. But they didn't stop locating the center of a woman's problems within her reproductive capabilities.

In the eighteenth and nineteenth centuries, hysteria was defined as any woman's unnatural proclivities for, as Rebecca Kukla notes in *Mass Hysteria*, "staying up late, attending the theater, taking up a profession."[11] The cure was to get married and have a baby. To rein in a woman, to stop her from deviating from the standard narrative, the fix was to control her body. Once married, once pregnant, a woman's body no longer belonged to her, but to her husband, her child.

It's no wonder we have not yet learned to untangle the problem of motherhood and depression, because we cannot see women as anything other than pathologized bodies and unstable minds.

The concept of "pregnancy brain" is one recurring narrative of mental instability in women. Pregnancy brain is the foggy thinking that people associate with pregnancy. The small studies that have been conducted have not been able to validate this phenomenon, but the myth persists. Maybe it's confirmation bias. Pregnant women expect to feel confused and disoriented, so they are.

I told a pregnant friend about the studies. She promptly replied that of course a man would make her feel like she was crazy by telling her she's not crazy. "My mind is different now," she said. "You can't convince me otherwise."

Is it real when we can measure it or is it real when a woman says it is happening to her?

When I was pregnant with my second child, I felt disconnected from the entire pregnancy. When he was born, I found myself still on edge, anxious and moody. After the day I screamed at my toddler daughter and then locked myself in my room, sobbing, while the baby cried, I asked my doctor for help.

My ob-gyn was a woman my mother's age, with three sons, who were all my age and younger. She was practical. No nonsense. That's why I liked her. With her, I did not feel pathologized. But her bootstrappy, just-figure-it-out approach to pregnancy had its flaws. When I told her of my exhaustion, my dark thoughts, my mood swings, she took out a medical text, turned to a section, and had me read it out loud. What it said was that no one knew what the effects were of antidepressants on nursing infants.

"You can have some if you want," she said closing the text. "Your choice."

Shamed, I said I was fine. I said I would control myself. I said I would try to sleep more.

I went home and told my husband. He said I had made the right choice. Four years later, in couples therapy, he would use that moment as evidence of my instability. I needed pills, I wasn't in my right mind.

After that, I went to my therapist, asking her—begging her—to tell me if anything was wrong, was I crazy? Did I need pills? Was I unstable? She reassured me I was a normal person experiencing a hard thing. She asked me what I thought I needed. What did I want? Turning it back on me, giving me the power over my mind.

Despite her reassurances, it was easier for me to believe I was losing my mind than to understand that I was losing my marriage. It's easy to gaslight a woman, after all. Tell her she just needs to try harder, sleep more. And then when that doesn't work, tell her she has failed. Tell her she needs to take care of herself, and when she tries, tell her it could harm her baby.

Depression is real. We know this. We know what it looks like and we have ways to treat it. But we make it so hard to access the treatment, or even the diagnosis. It can be nearly impossible to untangle it from our cultural baggage.

Like I said, it's not hard to gaslight a woman, just tell her that this is how it's supposed to be. *Rosemary's Baby* is terrifying to me because it's a reminder that women's perspectives are seen as less valid than men's, no matter how intimate and personal the subject.

I used to have an argument with my ex over another horror movie, *Hush . . . Hush, Sweet Charlotte*. When we watched the movie, I was shocked to see one of the characters die. "Is he really dead?" I asked.

"No," my husband said.

I waited the whole movie for the character to come back, but he never did.

"I thought you said he wasn't dead," I said.

"Yeah, I meant in real life."

That devolved into an argument about whether the actor playing the role had, in fact, died already. And another about whether the character being resurrected through a hallucination later in the film could be said to mean he wasn't dead. We went on like this until I was completely confused about all of it. We had the argument every time we talked about the movie, which was often, because I always felt like I was missing something. Like a game of mental "keep away" I wasn't big enough to win.

Throughout our twelve-year marriage, I kept coming back to it, wanting to settle it. I wanted to understand it. Understand what the hell he meant. What was he trying to pull? He never explained, not ever. Now that I've left, I cannot imagine we will ever return to that conversation. I know it was a joke to him, but it felt serious to me. I wanted to understand the terms of our conversation, whose reality were we operating in. What time period? Who got to define the terms of time and life and death? In so many ways, that fight felt like a microcosm of womanhood—a game in which someone is constantly changing the rules so you always lose. Maybe that's why I was so bothered by it. It never felt truly like a joke, but like a manipulation.

J. M. B., as we see in Tuke's case study, was a woman with few choices. She had to marry to be an acceptable woman. And with that marriage came birth after birth after birth. That is what society required of her. And yet each birth took something more from her. Was her madness her mind's resistance? Was it the result of long-untreated mental illness, made worse by lack of care, by the extreme waxing and waning of her body with each birth and the burden of caring for a growing family with little support?

It's not hard to imagine myself in J. M. B.'s place. Or in Catherine Linton's, staring in the mirror, haunted by reflections of a self I no longer recognize, a flesh rendered almost incomprehensible.

It's easy to gaslight a woman. Just tell her what she must do to be a good woman, a good mother, then give her a mirror.

Depths

On September 27, 1726, Mary Toft gave birth to a rabbit. She pushed it out of her vaginal canal, damp with her fluid. It was dead when it emerged, disemboweled and heavy—a strange lifeless mystery. It must have been a small rabbit, because some sources describe it as looking like a liverless cat.[1]

Mary was twenty-five and worked in a hops field. She couldn't read or write. Neither could her husband, who was a cloth worker, his job imperiled by industrialization. They were poor. They had had three children, though one had died as a baby. And Mary had had a miscarriage just the month before. But her womb was still swollen. She could still stroke the curve of her belly. Still imagine life within.

And then the rabbit came.

The next day, the town obstetrician examined Mary. When he arrived, her mother-in-law, Anne Toft, who had witnessed the birth, handed him the mutilated body parts of rabbits, which she said had been born during the night. That day, he watched as Mary birthed a rabbit's head, the legs of a cat, and nine dead baby rabbits. The accounts are shockingly detached. They note that the doctor "delivered" these parts or that Mary "procured" them. Soft verbs that obscure the process of birth. The screaming and the straining. The cries and the blood. The paw emerging from the red and raw lips of the vaginal canal. Fur mixing with hair mixing with blood. Her uterus contracted. The bed shook. The obstetrician was in awe. He wrote to everyone.

Mary went to London, where she birthed more skin, legs, ears, heads—raw flesh that added up to a whole rabbit. Sir R. Manningham, who witnessed one of the births, wrote that in the birth he observed her belly shook with the motions of the rabbit. The rabbits were leaping inside of her. But when they were birthed, they were dead.

It was a scam. She was found out mostly because a porter was caught bringing a dead rabbit to her room in London, where she lay, letting men pull rabbits out of her vagina. It didn't help that bits of hay were found in the fur of the rabbits she birthed. She went to jail but didn't stay there long. She'd fooled so many doctors and man-midwives, and they were ashamed. They sent her back to her home in Surrey, where she died decades later at sixty-two.

At the time Mary began having children, England was in the middle of a battle between midwives and the men who would supplant them—male midwives and doctors. Acceptance of male midwives was spread by Louis XIV's mistress Louise de la Vallière, who used a man midwife for all her births, and their social cachet grew. This was the start of the slow creep of patriarchal medicine into the process of birth. Male physicians and surgeons argued that midwives were provincial and unclean. Midwives argued men knew nothing about women and their inner workings. Male midwives were the in-between. They had gleaned the knowledge of midwives but exuded an air of science and that specific ethos of maleness. They also charged more money.

The argument for male midwives and physicians is that they did a lot to demystify the birth process. The eighteenth-century Scottish obstetrician William Smellie turned women's bodies inside out, enabling him to create anatomically correct and precise plates of a pregnant womb. But these male midwives and physicians could only observe so much about the process of pregnancy and birth, not experience it themselves, and I'm very wary of lauding men for the discovery of processes and interventions that were developed through experimentation on the bodies of women. Also, who's to say that women wouldn't have made the same discoveries if they hadn't been boxed out of the medical field?

Men entered the birthing room, approaching labor from an interventionist perspective, and were far more likely to penetrate a pregnant body with tools and medical implements. Intervention in birth as a policy would lead to an increase in maternal deaths due to infection and blood loss. Crucially, male practitioners also kept traditional midwives barred from medical practice. Rather than seeking to use the knowledge midwives had honed through generations of experience, they suppressed it.

Like early midwives, early male doctors and male midwives or male birth attendants were unlicensed and untrained. Some were dentists, and others were snake oil salesmen looking for another revenue stream. In *Get Me Out*, Randi Hutter Epstein recalls how in Victorian-era America, doctors often delivered a baby without even looking at the birth canal.[2] A sheet hung between the woman and the doctor as the doctor fumbled around for the child. One of my favorite images shows a male doctor on his knees in front of a woman, his hand up her skirt. He is examining her without seeing anything, and she is looking away, ostensibly out of modesty, but it's not hard to read a look of exasperation on her face as a man examines her without seeing her. An apt metaphor and a horrifying reality.

Two reports published in 1910 and 1912 show the extent to which American obstetricians were failing their patients.³ Ironically, the response to these reports would effectively cut midwives out of the birthing process. In a panic, politicians began to regulate birthing practices. A confluence of government paternalism and the capitalist enterprise drove advertising campaigns urging women to give birth in hospitals, where men, because of their access to higher education, reigned supreme. In 1915, 40 percent of all births were attended by midwives. By 1935, that number had decreased to little more than 10 percent. Midwives found themselves relegated to delivering in rural areas outside of hospitals.

There is a prevailing tendency in America to view the ascendancy of doctors over midwives as a triumph of modern science. But nothing could be further from the truth. For most of early American history, midwives came over from Europe as highly trained, well-respected professionals, or they were enslaved women who had been trained in their home countries and who trained later generations of enslaved women. And yet, as medical school training advanced and women were locked out of education, the gap in perceived legitimacy between male and female practitioners widened.

Men succeeded in bringing births out of the home and into hospitals, where infection raged—their intrusive and unwashed hands killed women in a careless epidemic. In 1866, a quarter of the women who gave birth in the Matemité Hospital in Paris died. Adrienne Rich writes in her classic *Of Woman Born*, originally published in 1976, about women running away to give birth rather than going to a lying-in hospital, where they knew they would likely die.⁴

But all of that came after Mary. She lay on the tipping point. The design for the first forceps would be revealed a mere fifty years later in 1773. Smellie would make his plates in the next century. When Mary "birthed" her rabbits, man was still groping his way around in the dark. Mary and women like her still gave birth in their homes. But men were making moves to take over medicine. And she, Mary, fooled many of those early physicians who formed the foundation of the practice of medicine as we know it today, weaponizing their ignorance of her body.

In 2019, my daughter wants to learn more about the body, her body. I buy her books detailing the body's organs. I buy a small skeleton, with organs and muscles. We sew bladders made from felt, watch YouTube videos of kidneys. The skeleton I bought has no reproductive organs. We discover this when she mistakes the liver for the uterus. We talk a lot about the different holes, what they lead to. But the mystery of inside of her remains. I wanted this cheap little skeleton, with its rubber organs, to help her put the pieces together. Instead of demystifying bodies, its makers decided to pretend that crucial organs that fill her abdomen don't exist. Of course, the vas deferens and penis and testes were also omitted, but that lack, while silly, isn't as gaping. The penis and scrotum make their presence known daily. The uterus and ovaries are buried deep inside. And in either case, divorcing children from their own bodies because of squeamishness is not in anyone's best interest.

Frustrated, I use Google for pictures. I'm trying to explain to her what's inside. I want her to have full control of her body. Knowledge is power.

Early Paleolithic societies honored the mystery of the female body in cave art. This period, the Aurignacian, is exemplified by drawings and images of women that emphasize their hips and breasts. The interior of the earth reflecting back the interior of the woman. In the Middle East, ancient tombs were designed as dark, spiraling hallways to mimic the interior of the female body, from which the dead could be reborn.[5] It's the earth as mother once again. In the places we can't see, seeds turn into plants and eggs into humans. Those moments happen out of sight, internally.

It makes sense, then, that men believed a rabbit could come from a woman's womb. I don't blame them too much. I know men in 2019 who still can't find the clit, and that's on the outside. The manifold mysteries of the reproductive system persist, even for women themselves. In 2016, a survey conducted by the Eve Appeal, a UK-based nonprofit that raises money for gynecological cancer, found that 44 percent of women were unable to identify the vagina on an anatomical diagram.[6] Sixty percent were also unable to identify the vulva.

The UK study resonates across Western culture. In Emma L. E. Rees's book *The Vagina*, she notes that vulvas are not depicted in art and in culture as often as penises. And when they are, they may be divorced from the female body, seen as dangerous.[7] Our culture is one of swinging dicks and hidden clits. We don't teach young girls to properly name the parts of their sexual anatomy, instead referring to it all as one thing—"a vagina."

Once, after I had my second child, I was at a child's birthday party. Two kids in tow, I was tired and sitting on a couch, letting my oldest, who was three at the time, play with her friends. A concerned mother came and sat next to me. "You should know," she said in a whisper. "Your daughter is telling everyone you 'pooped out a baby.'"

"I know," I said. "I keep telling her the baby comes out of the vaginal canal, not the rectum, but she will not believe me."

The mother stood, clutching her wine glass, and walked away. I realized in her retreat that her horror wasn't about the mislabeling of the vaginal canal but about the frank discussion of physical realities. The inability to name a thing disappears it from our consciousness.

For Mary, her power lay in this darkness. But for so many women, this lack of understanding creates chaos.

On Good Friday in 1276, Countess Margaret of Henneberg gave birth to 365 children. The children were as small as mice. Legend holds that half the children were girls and half were boys. The boys were baptized as Jan, the girls as Elizabeth. The sex of the odd-number child would be heavily debated. Some theologians (who were seen as authorities on all mysteries then) decided that that child was a hermaphrodite, just to make things even. Regardless, all those tiny children died, and so did their mother.

There are variations on this story. In one version, the countess had insulted a woman with quadruplets. In another, she insulted a woman with twins, making the father of the twins believe that his wife had cuckolded him; he placed his wife in jail until the countess gave birth to her 365 children, proving his beloved's innocence.

But all the stories follow the same pattern: a haughty rich woman insults a poor mother, and as a result, she is cursed with children—365 of them, all tiny fingerling babies, who die and take their mother with them.

Pieter Kaerius made an engraving of the scene of Margaret giving birth. It depicts a busy bedchamber, with Margaret in a canopied bed attended by a midwife. In the foreground, women boil water and busily minister the other tasks of birth. You might miss the 365 little bodies in a basin on a table in the far-left corner. They stand unnoticed and unattended. When I first saw those babies just standing there, I laughed. The absurdity is remarkable. Does no one care about these little babies? Is it better just to dip them in holy water and turn away?

The legend, of course, is dubious. But Margaret of Henneberg was a real person. Born in 1234, she was married to Count Herman von Henneberg. She had two children who survived into adulthood, a son, Poppo, and a daughter, Jutta. And she did die on Good Friday in 1276 at the family castle in Loosduinen, a small village in the Netherlands.

The first mention of Margaret's many children is in a late-fourteenth-century document that states simply, "During Easter, Countess Margaret of Henneberg gave birth to 364 sons and daughters and died quietly, together with them." From there, the legend grew until it reached an apex in the early seventeenth century. Childless women would travel to the Loosduinen Abbey and wash their hands in the basin that allegedly baptized all 365 babies. Of course, it wasn't the actual basin, if one had been used at all, if the babies had ever been born in the first place. But in matters of faith and miracles, proximity is more important than precision. And Margaret's curse would be their blessing.

Some sixteenth-century writers alleged that one of Margaret's children was preserved as a curiosity. The child was kept in the Kunst-kammer, the large cabinet of curiosities owned by King Frederick III of Denmark. One observer of the Kunst-kammer wrote about seeing a child, preserved in a glass bottle, hanging from a golden chain. He described it as black, with small white nails and as long as one joint of a finger.[8] In his book, *A Cabinet of Medical Curiosities*, Jan Bondeson surmises that the child in the Kunst-kammer must have really been the product of an abortion, passed off as one of Margaret's cursed children.

The legend of Margaret of Henneberg fell out of popularity in the seventeenth century, when one of the doctors who had given credence to the story of Margaret of Henneberg, John Maubray, was discredited after his gullibility in the scandal of Mary of Toft. Everything he believed was cast into immediate doubt, and the truth about Margaret of Henneberg became another casualty in the fight between science and myth.

As science continued to advance, her story had a renaissance in the 1930s when two doctors posited that her miraculous birth could have been the expulsion of a hydatidiform mole. A hydatidiform mole is a kind of mass that can grow inside the uterus. Inside the mole are cysts held together by thin strands of fibrous tissue. The children, the doctors speculated, were the cysts, spilling from her vagina like grapes falling out of a bag.

Whatever it was, it killed her.

The quasi myths of Mary's and Margaret's births are the inverse of each other. For Mary, the medical field's ignorance of her body was her power. She used it to scam people, quite successfully, for a time. But for Margaret, the mysteries inside her meant death.

This lack of knowledge still kills women. A 2017 investigation by ProPublica found that the United States has the highest maternal death rate in the developed world and that, of those deaths, a staggering 60 percent are preventable. The report traces the cause of these deaths to a healthcare system that focuses on the fetus more than the mother. Its authors, Nina Martin and Renee Montagne, note, "The growing specialty of maternal-fetal medicine drifted so far toward care of the fetus that as recently as 2012, young doctors who wanted to work in the field didn't have to spend time learning to care for birthing mothers."[9]

Preventable maternal deaths disproportionately occur to women of color, who face doctors and algorithms steeped in racial bias and who are rarely acknowledged as experts on their own bodies.[10] In Dr. Tressie McMillan Cottom's book *Thick*, she describes the traumatic birth and death of her daughter. She repeatedly told the doctors of her pain, which turned out to be preterm labor, and she was repeatedly dismissed. Cottom, a successful academic and writer, found herself deemed incompetent to know her own body by the medical establishment. Even tennis superstar Serena Williams nearly died because of complications following the birth of her daughter when her doctors didn't take her concerns seriously. For black women, class and credentials can offer only limited protection from the systemic racism in the medical establishment. As Cottom writes, "The assumption of black women's incompetence . . . supersedes even the most powerful status cultures in all of neoliberal capitalism: wealth and fame."[11]

Splitting the pregnant body into pieces allows these parts to be controlled, to become the domain of the medical establishment. We base expertise on clinical observation at the expense of personal experience, making adversaries of pregnant people and their doctors. And complaints of troubling symptoms are deemed normal or are dismissed entirely.

To me, and as others have described, pregnancy felt like an invasion. I chose the medical route. I was, after all, educated and "enlightened." Better living through science was my motto. As a result, the birth process felt more akin to the chest-burster scene in the 1979 movie *Alien* than to nature's miracle of life.

In 2019, the rapper T. I. bragged that he had doctors check his daughter's virginity. He later apologized and said he was mostly joking. But the comment sparked international outrage. At its core, the outrage was centered on the cultural misunderstandings of a woman's body and the protective paternalism that values one part of a woman over her whole.

It's the oldest trick in the book. Divide a woman against herself. She'll be so busy trying to hold herself together, she won't have time to do anything else.

Fathers like T. I. would deny this is their intent. Doctors, likewise, are often unaware of the cascading consequences of the assumptions and practices they learned in their training. But conscious or not, this logic creates a trap that our bodies fall into. Doctors do know a lot about our bodies, but so do we.

Centuries of medical knowledge have insisted that we know so much about the process of life. The images, the confidently detailed drawings in medical textbooks. What I tell my daughter is that, despite all of this information, there is still mystery, there are still unknowns, because a body is a complex organism, not discrete bits that add up to a mother and child. And in that space of dissonance between the parts and the whole, we have to make our own choices.

It's not that I want her to distrust doctors specifically. I just want her to distrust anyone who would take away her autonomy.

In March 2019, a news story told of a woman in Bangladesh who had given birth to a baby boy and returned to the hospital a full twenty-six days later complaining of stomach pain. It turns out she was in labor with twins, carried in a second uterus. The doctors had missed the two other babies, the extra organ, when she delivered the first. The story went viral, with people expressing both wonder and horror. It's a reminder that the days of Mary Toft are not behind us—the depths and darkness of the female body still contain mysteries.

For Margaret of Henneberg, like so many other pregnant people, the mystery of the uterus led to her death. Even for Mary of Toft, her uterus was a site of vulnerability. As a poor woman, children were extra mouths to feed. Pregnancy and birth were physically taxing and dangerous. Every time, she could die. Every time she gave birth, she was out of work for the lying in, losing out on income her family desperately needed. She turned her vulnerability into a moneymaking scheme. And it worked, too, for a while. Inside of her, in her darkness, lay her power.

Joseph Campbell wrote in *The Hero with a Thousand Faces*, "There can be no doubt that in the very earliest of ages of human history the magical force and wonder of the female was no less a marvel than the universe itself; and this gave to woman a prodigious power which it has been one of the chief concerns of the masculine part of the population to break, control and employ to its own ends."[12] If the history of birth is the story of men and medicine slowly taking over control of the female body, the story of Mary Toft is the story of a woman who twisted that narrative, just for a moment.

Part III

THIRD TRIMESTER

Your baby is now a butternut squash. Your baby is a cabbage. A pineapple. A head of romaine lettuce. Soon your baby will be a watermelon. And that watermelon will have to squeeze out of a hole the diameter of a small grapefruit.

You will take the birthing classes. The instructor will show you the various implements—vacuum, forceps—for removing that baby watermelon from your body. *Why not a shoehorn?* you will joke with your partner, who will not joke at all. They will want to focus. To make sure you know how to breathe, how to push, how to time your contractions. You will want to eat Taco Bell.

You will cry in the parking lot. You will cry eating breakfast sandwiches. You will know they are no good for you, but fuck that and fuck the watermelon, who is punching and kicking you. Pain will shoot up your crotch. You will google it. Somewhere on the internet a woman calls this lightning crotch. This will be funny. This will be sad. You will have lightning in your crotch. Why don't they tell you this? Why doesn't anyone tell you this?

"I'm tired," you will say to women, because you are so large you cannot get comfortable and your hips hurt and your legs hurt and you think you are dying, though you're not. Or maybe you are. You don't know. But you are tired. And the women will laugh and say, "Wait until the baby comes; you'll be more tired then." You will want to punch them. You will want to punch everyone. Especially the man at the hardware store who tells you that you make walking look difficult. Or the barista who frowns when you order a coffee. The women who reach out for your belly, your body, who stroke it without warning. Who tell you this is precious. Who tell you to savor it. Who get tears in their eyes while you are in the checkout aisle in Target and your acid reflux is so bad you think you are having a heart attack. *Savor this*, you want to tell them, while kneeing them in the groin.

Just kidding.

You are Mother Earth. You are Gaia. You are the embodiment of life. Paint your round belly as a globe. Do a dance in a river. Get those really amazing pictures taken. You know, the ones where gauzy silk streams off of your naked pregnant body while you stand in a forest. You're just so connected to nature, you know? You are leaning on a tree. You are a lifegiving orb of goodness. You also really, really, really want a hamburger.

Maybe your partner holds your stomach in a loving way. You make a heart with your hands over your stomach. This is life. This is precious. This is everything you want.

Or is it?

Count the kicks. You worry about breech. About birth. About plans. About playlists. About packing. About who will be there in the delivery room. About your life. About what you are leaving behind. About your body. Will it survive? Will you survive? Will everything be okay?

It's hard to say.

Congratulations. Your baby is a watermelon.

Power

Rows of men in inky black suits stare down at the dissected body of a woman lying on the surgeon's table. Their faces are white, in sharp contrast with their black suits. Some lean on their hands. Some seem to be nodding off. Some are speaking with their neighbor. The white cuffs and collars of their starched shirts peek out at varying angles. They are watching a surgeon cut open a woman's breast.

There are thirty-four identified people in the painting, which takes up a whole wall at the Philadelphia Museum of Art. Only one of those thirty-four is a woman, the nurse, standing aside as the operation is under way. The woman on the table is also a woman, of course. But she's not named. She doesn't count.

The painting is Thomas Eakins's *The Agnew Clinic*, which was painted to honor Dr. David Hayes Agnew, the famed physician who attended President Garfield when he was shot. It was commissioned for Agnew's retirement from Jefferson Medical College in 1889. It's a masterpiece—a vivid painting that roils with the dark colors and busy bodies of learning. The shadows of men. And the brilliant, glowing, bloody body of a woman.

Women are always lying naked and severed in our idea of medicine. A woman's body is always the center of a man's disection.

The painting was made to honor a man. But when I look at it, all I see is the degradation and silencing of a woman. I see a woman cut to pieces while so many male eyes look on. When I first saw the painting in the museum, I was there to look around. I was alone. A man had just broken my heart, and I felt silly and foolish about it all. I was a grown woman. A mother. I had taken a chance at romance. We'd gone on a road trip, had a fling, and he'd abruptly ended it all when we reached our destination. The reason was me, he said, my busyness, my children. I felt so silly. Women who pee when they sneeze don't usually get to do flighty, romantic things. But I'd done it. And it was over. Then, on a different trip two months later, trying to work, I was stripped naked of my context and again alone. I was sad, and craved my children. Their presence gives me purpose. In that museum, without a partner, without my kids—I struggled to understand how to live without someone looking at me, expecting something of my flesh.

When I had arrived at the Philadelphia Art Museum, the steps were filled with men and women taking pictures of themselves while making triumphant, raised-fist gestures. I was confused about why everyone was doing that, but happy for them. They all seemed to have something to celebrate. I texted a friend about it. She wrote back, "That's from *Rocky*, stupid."

Let me explain: I was homeschooled. I was raised without a television and missed out on a lot of cultural milestones. While many of my siblings and friends who were raised similarly worked to catch up later, I didn't. Not for sports movies, anyway. In college, a professor gave me a cultural dictionary, which I read like it was my new Bible—trying to learn the codes, the shared language of *Simpsons* quotes and John Hughes movie references, so I could fit in.

At some point, I got tired and quit caring. And I had never cared about *Rocky*. A movie about people punching each other in the face didn't make sense to me. So, I missed it. I missed that workout montage when Rocky dances at the top of the steps of the Philadelphia Art Museum, fists raised in triumph. I didn't understand, until I came face-to-face with it, that the gesture is a celebration of the male body.

I walked up those stairs into the museum and wandered around, looking at the idealized versions of women and children, until I happened upon the Eakins. There it was. It felt like looking at a crime. The violent triumph of one body over another. A woman bleeding. Men all around her, eyeing her, judging her, appraising her only as the work of the man, the surgeon. She doesn't even have a name. I sat down and cried. I had found myself in her position.

We are taught to believe in the supremacy of science, to celebrate the men of modern medicine. Barbara Ehrenreich and Deirdre English write in *Witches, Midwives, and Nurses* that it's a myth "fostered by conventional medical histories . . . that male professionals won out on the strength of their superior technology. According to these accounts, (male) science more or less automatically replaced (female) superstition—which from then on was called 'old wives tales.'"[1]

I had certainly bought into this idea for both of my pregnancies. After all, if this was the tried and tested way, why should I resist? I didn't need to be difficult. I didn't need to cause a fuss. I could just hand myself over to the professionals. I could trust them to do right by me. After all, it was science. It was dispassionate. It was not ruled by the whims of culture. Or so I believed.

Ehrenreich and English argue that in the early Middle Ages, before the expansive reach of the Catholic Church, birth was the realm of the mother and her community. Little is known about the actual experiences of midwives in antiquity, because so few women wrote the texts that inform our histories. But from medieval medical texts historians have inferred that midwives were professional healers, who treated manifold problems related to reproductive organs in addition to assisting with births. During the Dark Ages, this idea collapsed along with the cities that had served as intellectual centers, and the job of midwifery fell to groups of laywomen, neighbors, and relatives. Medical knowledge no longer relied on individuals but on the collective brain trust of the community—spanning the space between practice and belief, remedy and miracle. The work of these birth attendants, informed by experiential and instinctual knowledge, had enormous spiritual significance: the life or death of mother and child. As the Catholic Church grew in power and strength, midwives came under scrutiny by church officials, who considered them a threat.

One of the few stories we have today of midwives in the Middle Ages is an apocryphal myth about Salome, one of the midwives who attended the Virgin Mary during birth. Salome had doubts about Mary's claims of virginity and went to check her after the birth. As soon as she saw the proof (whatever it was) of Mary's veracity, her doubting hand shriveled and was only restored after she apologized to the infant savior. In the story of Salome, faith and medicine collide. Salome sought medical knowledge and was rebuked. And yet, her search for knowledge gave credence to Mary's virginity. The ambivalence toward scientific investigation in the story of Salome demonstrates the extent to which early medicine was entwined with religious devotion. Salome seeks proof like a scientist and finds it, but she suffers for it.

Still, in this place between myth and science, midwives have reigned, often serving both as healers and religious leaders.

Ehrenreich and English describe how in medieval Europe people who could heal were seen as having been imbued with a divine gift. The presence of midwives threatened the very core of the church, which sought to control access to the divine. So, men rewrote the narrative of the midwives' power. If they could heal, it was because they communed with Satan, not the Lord. No longer spiritual healers, midwives became witches. Ehrenreich and English contend that, in the late fifteenth and early sixteenth centuries, midwives in Western Europe were "a political, religious, and sexual threat to the Protestant and Catholic churches alike, as well as the state."[2]

Further separating women from divine power, the medieval Catholic Church taught that, just as the savior was implanted into the Virgin Mary by the Father, a child was deposited into the mother by its father as a "homunculus," a fully formed human with a soul, one who bore no attributes of the mother. The homunculus was not safe until it again reached the keeping of men—the priest who performed the baptism ritual, sanctifying and cleansing the child.

As midwives were persecuted and outlawed, the men of the church stepped into the role of healer, though they had little to offer but empty prayers. In nineteenth-century French historian Jules Michelet's book *Satanism and Witchcraft*, on the history of witchcraft, he details the effects of this shift: "On Sundays, after Mass, the sick came in scores, crying for help,—and words were all they got: 'You have sinned, and God is afflicting you. Thank him; you will suffer so much less torment in the life to come. Endure, suffer, die. Has not the Church its prayers for the dead?'"[3]

This sentiment is echoed today by opponents of universal healthcare. In her book *Strangers in Their Own Land*, Arlie Russell Hochschild writes about people in rural Louisiana who vociferously oppose what they term "socialized medicine" and state that the Lord will meet their needs.[4]

Though midwives persisted, in opposition to the church, during the Renaissance and the Age of Enlightenment, a new adversary once again pushed them to the margins. As scientific progress was codified into practice, medicine began to favor formal education, which was largely accessible only to men. Birth was put into the hands of male doctors, who treated pregnancies as medical abnormalities, little more than diseases to be cured. This was a natural next step in the sidelining of women from their births and bodies, rendering them unqualified, voiceless, and dependent on men's expertise.

In nineteenth-century America, midwives would find themselves fighting the same battle.

Midwifery in the United States is now largely the domain of white women, but that's a relatively recent development. Midwives have a deep history in this land; they existed in America long before the European settlers invaded. And for much of US history, black women delivered both white and black babies in their work as midwives. In black slave communities in the antebellum South, midwives were the epicenter of faith and healing. This practice of black midwifery continued into the early twentieth century, even as midwives occupied the lower levels of the medical hierarchy.[5] These "granny-midwives" were pillars of their communities. One notable example is the incredible Biddy Mason, a freed black woman who used her earnings as a midwife in Reconstruction-era Los Angeles to become one of the city's first real estate moguls and philanthropists. But as state and federal regulations were passed to ensure the safety of medical practice, midwives like Mason were forced to the margins.

Circulars were disseminated painting granny-midwives like Mason as unkempt, unprofessional, a danger to the fragile white women who used their services.[6] This myth, of the frail white woman, also has roots in Christianity. Early biblical teachings that surmise that black people are descendants of Ham, who was cursed by his father Noah, have been cherrypicked to justify slavery and other atrocities committed against the bodies of black and brown people. The myth posits that women of the pure and blessed races need to be protected from the machinations of the cursed. In *The Temple of My Familiar*, Alice Walker's narrator explains the staying power of this particular myth:

> They said the mother of their white Christ (blonde, blue-eyed, even in black-headed Spain) could never have been a black woman, because both the color black and the female sex were of the devil. We were evil witches to claim otherwise. We were witches; our word for healers. We brought their children into the world; we cured their sick; we washed and laid out the bodies of their dead. We were far from evil. We helped Life, and they did not like this at all. Whenever they saw our power it made them feel they had none.[7]

White women, adjacent to power, cemented their position by denying the power of black women. They did this through whitewashing the defining myths of motherhood. Mary is the mother of God. Mary is perfect. Mary is white.

Science, like the rest of human society, is not free from bias. And though it has brought us lifesaving vaccines and antibiotics and new understandings of our bodies, it has also, at times, failed us—particularly those of us who are women, trans, queer, people of color. And one of these times is birth. Birth is an incredible power, the only way to make new human life. And yet the experience of giving birth is so often one of powerlessness.

Modern birth stories often involve trauma from the loss of control that's become a standard part of the birth experience in the United States. Episiotomies, sedatives, surgical rupturing of membranes, forceps, the "vacuum"—all of these procedures are often forced on people giving birth. The expectation is that a good patient will passively accept whatever the doctor orders— and it always seems to be an order.

During my childbirth class at the hospital with my first, the nurse showed us the vacuum—a tool used to remove babies from the womb. I was horrified by how primitive it was. Just a tube that stuck to the baby's head and a kind of hand pump used for the suction.

"I hate that thing," I said to my husband. "I don't ever want it in me."

During birth, I pushed for four hours, and the doctor pulled out the vacuum. "I'm going to use this," she said. I wanted to object, but her tone left no room for discussion.

Everyone I talk to who's given birth has a similar story. Forced C-sections, medication they didn't ask for. Some women tell me about the "husband stitch," when the doctor sewing up a woman's vagina after an episiotomy adds an extra stitch to make her tighter for her husband, often without the woman's knowledge or consent.

The violence women experience during birth is nothing new. Margaret Mead wrote about it, as have Doris Haire, Brigitte Jordan, Adrienne Rich, and so many others, for over a century, and yet nothing has changed. Today, nearly a quarter of women who give birth report having PTSD symptoms afterward.[8]

Modern midwifery movements are trying to take back control of birth. But they, too, often miss the mark. A natural birth can be just as disempowering as a hospital birth. Rather than being just one option, it's positioned by proponents as the thing our bodies are made for, leading to a sense of failure if "natural birth" is not achieved. Natural birth isn't an option at all for many. It's often harder to find a doula or midwife than a doctor, and that level of care is inaccessible to the people who could benefit from it the most. Until we address income inequality or expand health-care access so people don't have to jump through hoops or pay out of pocket, homebirth, doulas, and midwives will be an option only wealthy, primarily white women can count on accessing.

Many advocates of the modern midwifery movement are call-ing for change, for better access to hospitals and better Medicare reimbursement rates. But change is slow. In Iowa, as rural hospi-tals close obstetrics units because of costs, the state is doing little to expand midwifery clinics. It's an easy solution that still faces strong-armed pushback from hospitals and physicians.

It has never truly been about who was in the delivery room, but about who was allowed to call the shots. It's about power and powerlessness. It's about class, race, gender, and who is allowed to speak for themselves (and for others). Over years of men con-solidating power, our personal choice—about sexuality, about birth control, about abortion, about giving birth—have been de-nied and made political. Our agency and our voices have been suppressed, silenced.

I grew up being taken to rallies protesting *Roe v. Wade*. I spent twelve years married to a man who believed abortion was mur-der. I have spent a good portion of my life (let's hope I live long enough so that it's not half my life) in churches where abortion was treated as a sin. So, I've heard the usual argument, the claim that the most vulnerable person in the room is not the woman, but the baby. The baby is the voiceless one. Who will speak for that baby?

The thing is, the whole premise of that question is bullshit. It creates a divide where none exists. Birth isn't about saving a baby from the person whose body has been sustaining and nurturing it, even at their own expense. It's about a person bringing new life into the world. The only relevant voice in that room is the pregnant person's. They are the one who chooses. They are the only one who can speak on their own behalf and that of their body. Their desires are not in opposition to the baby's but are part of creating that new life. To ask who speaks for the baby is to force a question where no question exists. It is to privilege the voice of another—a culture that wants the pregnant person to have less sex, be less poor, less black, less queer, less disabled, just less.

Changing the experience of birth requires changing the questions we ask. To do so, we must, as Adrienne Rich writes, "change women's relationship to fear and powerlessness, to our bodies, our children; it has far-reaching psychic and political implications."[9]

Recently, I met a friend for coffee. She has a three-year-old son and another on the way. She's exhausted. "A man is always grabbing at my body," she tells me. "If it isn't my doctor, it's my son, or my husband." She describes how she turns on the news and is flooded by stories of male lawmakers making decisions about her lives and small deaths. She's had an abortion. She's had miscarriages. Now she has these sons. I know how she feels. News story after news story breaks with news about a new law passed about birth control, about healthcare, about abortion. It's an assault, a power grab.

But the power lies naturally within us. It must make them feel so small that they don't have it. That they can't have it.

In 2017, the Trump administration convened a committee to discuss maternity healthcare coverage in the United States. A photo from the meeting shows a group of white men in suits, all gathered around a table to discuss the future of female bodies. The picture evokes the Eakins. It shows us powerful men making history. But what's not pictured, who is not named, speaks even louder. I look at the photo and see a message about the pow-erlessness of woman in a room full of men dissecting her body.

At a party, I tell a man who is a doctor about Eakins, and he tells me that's not what the picture is about. It's about honoring a man who contributed to medicine. "Women," he tells me, "are always so sensitive about these things." Always misunderstanding the situation.

He's right. That's the narrative of the picture. But that's the trouble with these pictures: they are always telling the wrong story.

Pain

I am the only woman here by herself on this serial killer tour of Philadelphia. Everyone is coupled up. A lesbian couple, a mother–daughter pair, three friends who seem like academics— but maybe it's just the turtlenecks they're wearing—and two heterosexual couples.

"Is it just you?" the tour guide asks me.

"Yup."

"So, just the one?"

"Yes, all alone!" I shout back. Everyone stares. I square my shoulders and smile. I want to be brave and fun and free. But the reality is, I am a woman alone on a tour of female pain. Our tour guide, Ted, hands out soft pretzels and small airplane-sized bottles of booze. I down a Fireball. And off we go.

The story of womanhood is the story of pain. It's been like this from the beginning, when Eve was cursed with pain in childbirth for eating that fruit.

I am on this tour because it sounded like fun, and I am in Philadelphia doing research anyway. I came to the city to look at the lying-in hospital and the Mütter Museum, where I saw relics of birth and bodies and babies. I've read the books about the men who wrenched the babies from the wombs, who preserved them in jars, who cut the mothers and opened them, and drew their insides, who are lauded as innovators. I saw the tools they invented for prying women open, for digging through their wombs, for grabbing, clawing, and scooping out babies from inside of them. I saw the babies themselves, small, broken bodies, preserved as monstrous anomalies.

But it's not until I am walking on this tour that I actually understand that everything I've seen is the story of pain. That the story of pain is the story of birth, as we often tell it.

Gary Heidnik is Philadelphia's most notorious serial killer. He kidnapped, tortured, and raped women, with the goal of getting them pregnant. He preyed on women who were marginalized, black, mentally disabled. His wife, who eventually left him, was a mail-order bride from the Philippines. Heidnik is the eighth person we learn about on the tour. We don't actually go to his house. Instead, we stop in Elfreth's Alley, a historic alley where little has changed in the last three hundred years. It's not a place any crimes took place, it's just a quiet place where the guide can tell every gruesome detail. The tour guide tells the Heidnik tale with lurid details, pausing as tour groups with young families walk by.

The previous stop had been at Betsy Ross's house. I had been excited to learn we were going there. Had Betsy Ross killed a man? No. Apparently, we stopped there simply to learn that the tour guide thought Betsy Ross was hot and had great tits. Then we walked on and learned about Heidnik in an alley where nothing has changed, and it couldn't have been more perfect, because truly nothing has.

The field of obstetrics was built on women's pain at the hands of men. Specifically, in the United States, the pain of enslaved black women. J. Marion Sims, known as the father of American gyne-cology, experimented with the speculum and the fistula-repairing technique that would make his name on enslaved women whose names have been forgotten—without anesthesia. The techniques used in obstetrics today were fine-tuned on the bodies of women of color, in brutal experiments that killed many, many women. More than Heidnik ever did.

Sims's defenders argue that he was just adhering to standard medical practice at the time. It's a damning defense: he killed black women because everyone was killing black women. This defense implies, rightly, that many of our medical advancements were built on the pain of black women. From the Tuskegee exper-iments to the cells of Henrietta Lacks, medicine established itself on the bodies of the disenfranchised.[1] And there is a cost beyond the invisible body count (which should in itself be enough): rac-ism was encoded into our healthcare system. When black bodies are not being used as test subjects without their consent, they are denied care or are given inadequate care.

The story of American obstetrics today is the same as when Sims ripped apart all those black women's bodies.

One of the assumptions Sims and his colleagues made about black bodies was that they were somehow inured to pain. They didn't feel it. It's a myth that persists to this day. As a result of racial bias and this history of racist assumptions, black patients are more likely than white patients to be undertreated for pain.[2]

These days in the United States, someone in labor can gen-erally choose whether to have an epidural to block the pain of childbirth, but for a long time that pain wasn't seen as something any woman should be able to get relief from. In colonial Amer-ica, childbirth pain was fetishized. After all, their foundational myths told them pain was Eve's punishment, her daughters' bur-den to bear. A husband's role was to sit beside his laboring wife and read scripture to her, to remind her that woman had brought this on herself. As if that was any sort of comfort.

In Martin Luther's 1522 work, "The Estate of Marriage," he writes:

> This is how to comfort and encourage a woman in the pangs of childbirth, not be repeating St Margaret legends and other silly old wives' tales but by speaking thus, "Dear Grete, remember that you are a woman, and that his work of God in you is pleasing to him. Trust joyfully in his will, and let him have his way with you. Work with all your might to bring forth the child. Should it mean your death, then depart happily, for you will die in a noble deed and in subservience to God."[3]

This was the "thoughts and prayers" approach to childbirth for centuries. What little we know of midwifery at the time tells us that midwives also told women their pain was not just inevitable, but also the curse of the divine. And the women giving birth viewed it as such, too. In preindustrial America, childbirth was just one of many potentially fatal threats women faced. Every trial was borne with the knowledge that pain was the result of the Fall, a consequence of a woman's sin.

As the craft of medicine began to take over childbirth, men began to play God. The first doctor who administered a pain reliever to a woman in birth was James Young Simpson. The Scottish doctor used chloroform on another doctor's wife in the late 1800s. In Simpson's biography, his daughter recounts that the mother was so delighted, she named her daughter Anaesthesia. In reality, that was Simpson's nickname for the girl who had been baptized "Wilhelmina." Regardless, the Scottish church was less pleased, arguing that Simpson's methods were tools of Satan.[4]

That belief has a long history. In 1591, a woman in Scotland was sentenced by King James VI to be burned alive as punishment for general witchery, which included drinking a potion that she believed would bring her pain relief during labor. The midwife who gave it to her was also sentenced to death, as a witch.[5] A woman attempting pain relief was a woman subverting God's will.

Some doctors continued to oppose using anesthesia, but their concerns were based more in bias than in biology. Charles Delucena Meigs of Philadelphia argued in the mid-1800s that a woman should labor in pain because it made her love her child more. This twisted logic persists today and can be heard when women speak of feeling more bonded to their child because of the pain of delivery.[6]

In the early twentieth century, some US feminists fought to end suffering in childbirth. It felt revolutionary to fight for pain relief, after centuries of men telling you you should just take it. Just deal with it, all because you were born a woman. All because a man put his dick in you and you, having no access to reliable birth control, got pregnant. If the very least you could do was not scream in agony every time you risked your life to birth one of those children, well then, that was something. Actually, it was everything. It was a way to push back against the curse.

Their offer of salvation came from Dr. Joseph DeLee of Chicago, who in 1920 made the case against a natural approach to birth, arguing that it damaged both mother and baby. DeLee proposed a series of medical interventions, including forceps and sedatives, to protect women from the "evils natural to labor."[7] Women, wealthy white women in particular, eagerly embraced this approach to birth. The *Ladies' Home Journal* ran articles touting "twilight sleep" as a cure for the "primal curse." Thus twilight sleep, a method of birth that involved completely sedating a mother during delivery and that could only be carried out in hospitals, was championed by early-twentieth-century feminists. (It's worth noting that these same feminists advocated for the creation of nursing as a profession, which subjugated a whole class of women to a secondary role in their own healthcare.) But it was a Faustian bargain. What had seemed like freedom from pain and from the patriarchy of the oppressive Christian myth was subjugation of another kind.

In sum, pain-free births looked like a way for women to retake control of their bodies, but in choosing that option they gave up the ability to make other choices for themselves. In embracing twilight sleep, women surrendered themselves to a system that rendered them powerless and built a medical practice on their subservient, drugged-up bodies. Even today, when pregnant people are conscious during labor, they often struggle to resist medicalized procedures. Someone who wants to refuse a sweep of their membranes or an unnecessary C-section must fight against the pull of the system, and even then, their wishes are often ignored or forgotten. It's telling that many pregnant people feel they need to hire doulas as birth advocates to help their voices be heard. Upper-class white women, of course, are most likely to have doulas. They're the ones who can afford them. Those who can't have to hope for the best.

The push for pain-free births fed into the narrative of frail white women who needed to be protected. Who needed a man to put them at ease and deliver their baby for them. Birth was complicated, after all; let the doctors handle it. So women did. And the promised pain relief rendered them inert, powerless, further handing birth over to the medical establishment.

Later, in the 1960s and 1970s, women wanted to reclaim their power and their role in birth. As a result, when women began to push back against overmedicated births, pain was reclaimed.

This time, pain wasn't subjugation, pain was freedom. Birth was beautiful. Women no longer wanted to be objects—passive observers in the births of their children. They wanted to be active in the experience of their bodies. Pain became noble again. It had a purpose. But that wasn't liberation either. Once again, a woman's value was tied to the suffering of her body.

Three months after I gave birth to my first child, my husband told me that birth hadn't hurt me that much. He'd overheard me telling a friend about the epidural and the hemorrhaging, how my doctor wouldn't tell me how many stitches I'd been given, how I was still crying from pain when I pooped.

"It wasn't that hard," he said. "You got an epidural and then read a book."

He was right. I did get an epidural and I did read *The Great Night* by Chris Adrian, tearing through the novel as if it was the last one I'd ever read. (And it was, for a while at least.) But the pain tore through. Epidurals don't result in painless births. They just mitigate the pain. And they wear off. In the aftermath of the birth, I was passing in and out of consciousness. I bled so much they had to bring in a surgeon to consult. Once, when I woke up, I saw a nurse mopping my blood off the floor. The bucket was red. "It's like the tide at Omaha Beach," I said, before passing out again.

The cruelty of his comment aside, it exposed the underlying belief that pain was de rigueur for my body. To be expected.

It's true, pain is in many ways a woman's default mode of being. When Mary Wollstonecraft died of sepsis, which she contracted while giving birth assisted by a male doctor in dirty conditions, the Reverend Richard Polwhele remarked that her early death was her fate as a woman: "She died a death that strongly marked the distinction of the sexes, by pointing out the destiny of women."[8]

It sounds archaic, but it rings true even today. The United States has the highest maternal death rate in the developed world. If men died like this, at this rate, we'd declare a national emergency. But we don't; we expect women to die in childbirth. Adrienne Rich writes, "The identification of womanhood with suffering—by women as well as men—has been tied to the concept of woman-as-mother."[9]

In a poem titled "When God Created Mothers," written in 1974, Erma Bombeck exalts the idea of mother as pain vessel, describing God's efforts to create a mom with his angel sidekick. As God builds his prototype, the angel notices that the mom seems too soft. "But tough!" responds God excitedly. "You can imagine what this mother can do or endure."

Bombeck's poem endures because women identify with the idea of being someone who endures, who suffers.

Pain is how we expect women to walk through the world. Once, a stranger on the internet tweeted at me that he was sad for my children to have a mom like me. When I replied, countering that his comment was mean, he expressed surprise that I would respond, arguing that I was a "public figure" and therefore should just accept criticism.

Public figure, here, meant "woman on the internet." It meant, a person being a mother in public. It meant, just take it—this is your role, your inheritance. It fit into a familiar logic. Before that, once, when I told my husband about something mean someone had emailed to me, he had responded, "Isn't that what you get, writing like that?"

It's not hard to take that comment and turn it into: "Isn't that what you get, being dressed like that?"

"Isn't that what you get, being pregnant like that?"

". . . being born a woman like that?"

". . . being black like that?"

". . . being gay like that?"

". . . being trans like that?"

As if however we're treated is deserved, a reasonable punishment for our very existence. It goes back to Eve. Or, at least, back to how we read that myth. And that has tethered us to our pain.

In Iran, like in the United States, religion strongly influences the culture. Unlike in the United States, in Iran religion is state-sponsored—90 to 95 percent of Iranians are Shia Muslim, and religious observance is a strong cultural value. A 2015 study of childbirth practices in Iran found that many women chose nonmedicated, vaginal delivery because they saw it as a fulfillment of God's plan. The study's authors note: "Some of the pregnant women believed that natural birth is a holy phenomenon since one can praise God and get closer to Him. They believed that if the expecting mother died while giving birth, she could reach the sublime degree of martyrdom." The participants believed that if they endured labor pain, God would forgive their sins and therefore accept their prayer. They weren't alone in this belief. A researcher observed one of the midwives telling a woman in labor: "Please pray for whatever you want, now God forgives you and accepts your prayers, please try to pray for those who want a baby, pray for us, too."[10]

The embrace of "natural" childbirth as God's plan can also be seen among Christian groups in the States. The language of Evangelical groups such as "Alpha Childbirth," which is a childbirth education curriculum that endorses natural childbirth as part of the divine plan for women, echoes the language observed in the Iran study—encouraging a reliance on faith and prayer to endure the pain and complications of childbirth. The interchangeability of this rhetoric with the Shia rhetoric in Iran, and the contrast between it and other, more progressive Christian traditions, underscores the malleability of myth.

US culture in general glorifies the pain of motherhood, as it has since the Puritans settled here, even at the expense of women's health and welfare. Proponents of natural birth often play into this unhealthy ideal. Many women in the United States who planned to have natural childbirths and eventually had medical intervention have experienced overwhelming feelings of failure. Blogger Maria Guido wrote that she desperately wanted a "natural" childbirth, believing that her body was created for that purpose. Even after having to be induced at forty-one weeks, Guido refused medical intervention in the form of pain medicine. She finally agreed to a C-section when the doctor told her her son's heart was slowing and would soon stop. Afterward, holding her son, instead of feeling grateful, she felt distraught. The pain of failure followed her for several months. She had tried to do what she believed her body was uniquely created to do, and something went wrong. As Guido notes, both dogmas of birth—the natural midwife and the overly medical—fail to make room for the full, messy human experience of birth.[11] There has to be a better way and it has to begin with changing the stories we tell ourselves. Our pain has to be more than a curse. We must be worth more than our pain.

In the Netherlands, birth is a collaborative effort between the midwife and the person giving birth that is based on scientific inquiry into the country's birthing outcomes. There, knowledge is horizontal: midwives confer with their patients to make the best decisions based on a person's bodily needs. Contrast this to the United States, where birth is a medical procedure, and the pregnant person's choices and knowledge of their own body are subordinated to the superior knowledge of the doctor, the hospital staff, and the electronic monitors. When it comes to childbirth in America, knowledge is a hierarchy; although expectant parents are often encouraged to plan births according to their own opinions and personal preferences, their choices are respected only so long as they are convenient for the doctors, the dominant authority.

In the Netherlands, when a person is pregnant, their primary care physician refers them to a midwife for prenatal care. This prenatal care is covered under the country's universal healthcare, and checkups with the midwife are informal and relaxed. Before the birth, parents are often given kits called *kraampakket*, which include all the supplies necessary for a home birth. Doctors are involved only if the pregnancy is deemed high risk, and even then, this care is free at point of service. People can choose to deliver at home or in the hospital, and even in a hospital, the midwife delivers the baby.

In American hospitals, a person in labor must convince the hospital not to give them medicine. In the Netherlands, no epidurals or anesthetics are administered unless requested, because birth and its accompanying pain are seen as a natural process rather than a crisis situation to be mitigated with medicine.[12]

The ancient faiths practiced in the Netherlands blended Celtic, Roman, and Norse beliefs. One interpretation of a Norse legend posits that man and woman sprang to life from pieces of ash and elm. Unlike in Christian stories of creation, there is no male-gendered God as the orchestrator of all life. In Nordic myths, life is a creation of nature itself—men and women appear on the beach as wood before the gods, who impart to them spirit, mind, and blood. Celtic mythology is less clear on the origins of humanity. From the earliest Creed of the Celts, man is born of Earth and Heaven, along with the gods and the giants. Mixed up in a divine mess of blood and war and floods, we are there from the start, beholden to no one. In this violent world, there is no neat hierarchy, and gods and mortals spar as equals.

The Netherlands has more recent religious influences, too. During the sixteenth and seventeenth centuries, these played an important role in the Protestant Reformation. It was there that

Menno Simons became an Anabaptist leader whose followers would found the Mennonite church. It was William I, the first leader of the Dutch Republic, who in 1566 converted to Calvinism and in 1568 led a rebellion against the Catholic Church that resulted in the widespread embrace of the Protestant faith. But after World War II and the German occupation of the Netherlands, secularism slowly took hold. As a result, the Netherlands began to look like it had in its earlier history, when a polytheistic blend of faith and myth was the dominant creed. Today, these myths are mainly symbolic. But they are powerful, offering a vision of equality and the idea that the inception of life is as natural as driftwood on a beach.

The United States also has myths that belong to the rightful custodians of our land, before the religion of the Pilgrims and settlers infiltrated. For the people who hold fast to those stories as the organizing principle of their culture, birth is still seen as a natural occurrence. A 2003 study of Native American communities in New Mexico showed that even with higher rates of gestational diabetes and preeclampsia, Native American women needed less medical intervention in birth than the national average because of strong support systems and cultural attitudes toward birth. Settlers aggressively rejected these beliefs over the years, colonizing the land and converting, killing, or driving out Native Americans in a campaign of genocide. Despite the recent fetishism and appropriation of Native American art and clothes, US citizens continue, to our detriment, to resist understanding the culture and founding myths of the people whose land we occupy.

I do not demand that we erase Eve. I do not think we can forget her story. But I do think we can retell it. I think we can acknowledge her pain and honor it. And that begins by handing her pain back to her rather than inflicting it on her. That begins by allowing her to choose, which is, after all, what she did in the first place.

What if that is her story? Not one of malice or idle curiosity or impulsiveness, nor even arrogance. What if it is about choice? What if, when we tell that myth, we say that Eve knew, and she chose a full human life—one with pain and affliction, but also one with free will and children—over an easy Eden, where everything was handed to her and nothing was asked of her.

The curse isn't a curse, it's just our reality. The consequence of living a life of choice rather than a life chosen for us.

It's not hard to draw a line between Heidnik and our cultural attitudes toward women's bodies. When a recent study found men under thirty were having less sex than expected, Wikileaks responded that young men were being "deprived of romance" and children. As if women's reproductive capabilities were owed to anyone. As if our bodies were a man's birthright. As if our pain was of no consequence. As if our destiny were to be martyred for the advancement of humanity. Or of science. As if our blood and pain needed to be spilled for the good of all.

Walking the serial killer tour, with my whiskey and pretzel, felt like taking a kind of communion—a remembrance of the women martyred for the vitality of the city. We walked along to the soundtrack of story after story of women murdered. Philadelphia is an old city. Laying the foundation for anything new requires excavating old bones.

I am an avid consumer of crime. I watch *Forensic Files* and *Deadly Rich*; I listen to podcasts with names like "Crimetown" and "My Favorite Murder." I sign up for ghost tours and this serial killer tour. Walking with my bread and booze, I consume pain. I don't like this about myself. But I do it. Sometimes I wonder whether I seek out stories like this because I want to learn them and, in learning them, understand them as more than just pain.

Miracles

I went to Idaho in search of miracles. In the shadow of the Rocky Mountains, almost anything feels possible. The ancient monsters of rock boulder their way through the earth. The colors are surreal—violet shadows, cerulean shade, fuchsia skies.

Living here feels impossible. There are nineteen people for every square mile of land. Only six states in the United States can claim a more isolated landscape. With its deserts, deep canyons, and high mountains, much of this state is inhospitable and inaccessible.

When I pick up my rental car, the woman at the counter looks me up and down and asks where I am going.

Clifton, I say.

"You need a truck," she says.

"It's okay, I prefer a car."

She smiles and hands me the keys to a Ford F150. "Good luck."

It's not hard to drive to Clifton from the Idaho Falls Airport. Most people drive in from Salt Lake and I could have flown in through there. I'll spend the rest of my next three days in the state wondering if maybe I should have. Wondering if I haven't done absolutely everything wrong.

I'm in Idaho because I read a book. Specifically, *Educated*, the best-selling memoir by Tara Westover. Westover is the youngest of seven children, raised in Clifton by parents she describes as devout Mormon survivalists. She was homeschooled and struggled to get an education. She also describes the patriarchal structure of her home and the physical and psychological abuse she endured from her older brother. Westover now has a doctorate from Trinity College, Cambridge, and is estranged from her parents, Val and LaRee Westover, who deny she was abused and claim she has fallen away from the truth of God.

Years ago, Val, Tara's father, was severely burned in an explosion, and LaRee treated him at home with essential oils. *She* didn't heal him, she tells me on my second day there, *God* healed him. She just followed God's lead. LaRee had worked as a midwife for more than thirty years and has since retired. Now she runs a business selling essential oils out of their home in Clifton, where she also holds workshops and records YouTube videos and a podcast about oils and life and healing.

Val and LaRee don't think their daughter is lying; they think she's confused about the truth. They think she needs to come home, to remember who she is. While I am there, they pray for her at every meal and right before bed. They pray for me, too, that I will hear and report the truth of their life and their faith.

I am in Idaho because I want to understand mothers, and daughters, and families, and life, and miracles. Val and LaRee say that I am here because they prayed and the voice of God told them to let me come into their home.

Like Westover, I grew up homeschooled in a large family. And I also had parents who rejected medicine in favor of a blend of homeopathy and prayer, and we saw doctors only when absolutely necessary. We were Evangelical and lived in Texas, right outside of Dallas. When I was little, my mom would grind wheat for her bread, procure milk straight from a cow, and buy buckets of raw peanut butter from the co-op for us to blend with honey and smear over the thick slices of rough homemade bread. My parents' experiment in survivalism was relatively short-lived—by the time my youngest brother was born, my dad had gotten cable TV and my mom sent us older three to public school—but it was long enough to define my childhood.

I remember pressing my ear against the door of the living room while my parents watched the news on the TV they kept on a cart and rolled into a closet. The first newscast I actually watched, I saw at the home of family friends, who were watching us overnight while my parents went out on a date. The parents must have thought I was asleep, in my sleeping bag on the living room floor, because the TV was silent and all I saw was a building on fire and the muted panic of the journalists. Waco was burning. I thought the world was over. Later, I would hear my parents talk about David Koresh at after-church lunches of brisket and biscuits, when the children had been sent to play kickball outside. I would stay back to clean the kitchen just so I could listen to the men talk.

This is what I heard: The government would come for us if we were not vigilant. This was an attack on religion. On our freedoms.

During the school year, my mother instructed us not to answer the door during the day. When we were out, we were to tell people we went to a private school. A newsletter mailed to us by an advocacy group, the Homeschool Legal Defense Association, warned that we could be taken away from our parents at any moment by a power-mad liberal, secular government.

I am one of eight children, the second oldest. The family I grew up in was vastly different from the family my younger siblings grew up in. I remember measuring the hems of my shorts to make sure they were modest enough for camp and my mom sewing us jean jumpers with iron-on puff paint images of Holly Hobbie on the front. I remember long days playing with my siblings in the creek behind the house, where we used the junk the strip mall dumped from the overpass to make a little shantytown. We created our own system of government, our own rules, and even, thanks to my brother Zach and his meticulous attention to detail, our own currency.

But by the time I was in college, my family lived in a house in St. Petersburg, in Florida, just a short walk from the pier. Without me, my family spent days on the beach eating fried chicken. My sisters often acted as the rebels at the private religious school they attended—swearing, dyeing and cutting their hair, wearing two-pieces, and sneaking out to go drinking. Even though I was older and married by then, I would get nervous when they would do so much as turn on the TV to watch a cartoon.

"Does Mom know?" I'd ask.

They'd roll their eyes and continue watching *The Simpsons*.

I remembered my *Simpsons* pencil, a gift from a distant aunt, being confiscated when I was twelve. I had no idea it was a TV show until I went to high school. I hardly recognized this version of my family.

In the story of my birth, my mother says my father caught me. This detail is important. It casts me as my father's daughter. As she tells it, I was a very calm baby, except when I would freak out and sob uncontrollably. She tells me this story when—once a year, like clockwork—I call her to sob uncontrollably. I am easy until I am difficult. Calm until I am an ocean of unmitigated emotion. Our origin myths shape our stories.

But this is not the story I want to tell of my life. It's not the truth of who I am. I want a different myth.

I went to Idaho because, more than just understanding birth, I want to understand creation.

Every human birth feels like a miracle. A triumph of the impossible. Whereas most mammals can give birth alone, humans require assistance. The working hypothesis for this fact is known as the "obstetrical dilemma." The obstetrical dilemma is this: To stand upright, walk, and run requires humans to have a narrow pelvis. But to deliver our big-headed babies, we need a wide pelvis. These competing evolutionary forces created a bottleneck in the birth canal. This is why human birth is so painful, the hypothesis proposes. It's why we need cesarean sections and medical assistance: for the body of a human child, which is about the size of a watermelon, to be pushed out of the vagina, which is about the diameter of a lemon, the baby must be positioned so that the head can slip out first, or it will get stuck.

But maybe the obstetrical dilemma has it all wrong. Maybe this theory is ahistorical and biased and used to justify medical intervention and the pathologizing of the female body. Ancient images, from archaeological excavations in Europe, South America, and the Middle East, all show women giving birth alone in upright positions.[1] And some women still give birth like this today.

"Tell me why we need vaccines," Val challenges me on my first night in the compound in Clifton. We are sitting in the main room, with its high wooden ceilings, and there is a kitchen, a television, large comfortable couches, golden oak cabinets, tables, and chairs. The brown walls are lined with pictures: Joseph Smith, Jesus, a dove alighting from heaven, the Mormon Tabernacle at sunset.

"So we don't get polio," I say.

He frowns. "Money, it's all about the money."

LaRee gently pats his thigh. A warning.

"It's a global conspiracy. A Jewish conspiracy."

LaRee's pat turns into a squeeze and he stops.

According to a 2016 Pew Research Center study, only 17 percent of Americans distrust the scientific consensus on vaccinations.[2] But they are a vocal minority. In September 2019, anti-vax protestors marched on the California state capitol to oppose a law that would prevent parents from using religious exemptions to opt out of vaccinating their children. "No segregation, no discrimination, education for all!" they chanted, carrying signs that read, "Welcome to Nazifornia."

The anti-vax movement has found itself at the center of a weird Venn diagram of American culture. Religious fundamentalists, left-leaning hippies, movie stars, and conspiracy theorists are the strange bedfellows leading the movement.

It's not that they don't believe in science, LaRee explains the next morning, once we're all rested and Val has left to go check on the animals. They just believe in creation, in the body, in the ability of nature to heal. And have a deep distrust of the government.

After all, why wouldn't you? Nine hours away, near Naples, Idaho, is Ruby Ridge, the site where Randy Weaver, his family, and their friend Kevin Harris held out in an eleven-day standoff with the FBI that resulted in the deaths of Deputy US Marshal William Francis Degan, the Weavers' fourteen-year-old son, Sammy, Weaver's wife, Vicki, and the family dog.

We don't talk about Ruby Ridge. Instead, we talk about birth.

LaRee is a licensed midwife. She tells me she's delivered hundreds of babies. Her favorite story is the one about her grandson, who I'll call John. John's mother is married to the man Tara calls Shawn in her book—the brother she accuses of verbal, psychological, and physical abuse.

As LaRee and I talk, Shawn drifts in and out of the room. He doesn't speak to me, not directly, not ever, not even when we have dinner together on my last night there. He just stares at me.

As LaRee tells me the story of John's birth, Shawn interrupts to ask her where the funnels are.

"Funnels are in the second drawer in the corner. Drawer. Corner, where the whole row of drawers is."

She tells me how John's mother had fibroids and was told by a doctor to have an abortion. "She just stood up and walked out. Here she is, twenty-three years old, she gets up and walks out of the room. She was better taught than that."

LaRee had the doctor sign a piece of paper saying he'd advised an abortion. She didn't mean anything by it, she tells me. She just wanted reassurance. Later, after the baby was born and if the government tried to prosecute for child endangerment, LaRee would ask them if they could spell out child endangerment, because she spells it "abortion."

LaRee brought her daughter-in-law home from that initial doctor visit and prepared for the worst. The young woman made it to the twenty-seventh week—the last of the second trimester. John slid into the world in LaRee's back bedroom. It was a really horrible February day. The worst storm of the winter season that year. LaRee and Val had just come home from town. They almost stayed at LaRee's parents' house, but it didn't feel right. So they drove home, walked in the door, and her son explained that his pregnant wife had been bleeding for about two hours.

"What's this baby's chance of survival if we don't get this labor shut down?" Shawn asked.

"Slim. He's small for days. I don't think he's got a shot at it, hun." They cried, together.

"If we load her in the car and take her to town, we'd have a better shot there," Shawn said.

"Marginally," LaRee cautioned. The weather was too bad.

They made a plan to stay at the house as long as they could but to take her to town if it got too bad. She slept another hour, and when she woke up, she felt pressure. Not a contraction. Just pressure.

LaRee put on a sterile glove and checked her. What she felt was his tiny little head right there. She delivered him, and after twenty seconds she held him in her hand.

She had the training and the equipment. She breathed into his lungs. He was such a strong little spirit. She was standing there holding little John and her son was hugging his wife.

"They're crying and I'm saying to myself, 'Okay, do I hand him [over to them]? He's alive, he's so alive. Do they get to hold him when he's this alive? Then watch him die? Or would it be better for me to handle that?' About the time I'd completed that thought, this little voice in my ear says 'Grandma, I could use some help here.' Okay."

She pressed gently on little John's back, over and over, until she felt a little heart beating. Then she put him on his mother's chest. Later, they took him to the hospital, where LaRee visited him every day—holding him, doing energy work on him.

He was so small his arm could fit through a wedding ring, LaRee says. He weighed only twenty ounces. Due in the sunshine of July but born in a storm in February.

I have a hard time believing the story. I check it every which way. I call around to doctors' offices in Clifton and no one calls me back. I speak with one doctor who tells me, yes, the story sounds incredible, but plausible. I have no reason to doubt it, except that I feel like I have to.

My own family has a story like this—the story of my brother Noah's birth. He was born two months early, after my mom fainted at a Bible study. She was toxemic. My dad took her to the closest hospital, in Sioux City, Iowa. She was air-lifted from there to Sioux Falls, South Dakota, because the Sioux Falls hospital had a better NICU. My father said that the doctor gave him a choice: save my mom or save the baby. He told him to save both.

My brother Noah was so tiny, he could fit into the palm of my father's hand.

Every birth begins a new story. We start in the womb and spend our lives spiraling outward, pushed and pulled by the gravitational force of our mother's body. When I first began to publish my writing about my family, my mother stopped talking to me. Here is how I remember it: I wrote an essay about my sister's abuse by someone close to us; my mother told me I was wrong. She told me I didn't have the facts right. I told her I was going to tell the truth and she couldn't do anything about it. And then she told me nothing. I got a Facebook message from a friend of hers. Did I know what I was doing to my mother? Did I?

I don't remember replying. If I did, I am sure I wasn't polite.

In the beginning, all we know are our mothers. When each of my children was born, I felt like they were part of me, attached to my body. I would wake up in anticipation of their cry. Even now, I sometimes feel phantom kicks inside me. I wonder what it's like to have your creation rewrite the story? How did God feel in Eden? How does LaRee feel now? What happens when creation becomes creator, what happens when daughters become mothers, when our origin stories are questioned?

This story I am writing in this chapter might not feel like a story of birth. But it is the only story of birth I understand. The search for miracles, the search for our mothers, and the understanding of our own narrative. In her art installation *My Birth*, the artist Carmen Winant compiled over two thousand images of birth she found in books and pamphlets and magazines. The project was shown at the Museum of Modern Art.

On the website, she explains, "By having 2,000 photographs, the work asserts that there's no single way to read a narrative into the project. This could be a shared narrative that both collapses time, and also sort of points to the difference between kinds of experience."[3] That birth is always happening and yet, when it happens to you, it feels as if you just discovered it. Each birth is unique. And yet, birth is always happening.

In the book Winant published about the collection, she weaves together these found images with photos of her own mother giving birth. She explains that the impossibility of birth "opens up possibility. My preoccupations with dealing with birth stems from the fact that I cannot possibly deal with birth."[4]

Birth often feels impossible, whether because of the evolution of my pelvis and my child's head or because of a medical system that pathologizes my body and a culture that limits my choices, criminalizing them or making them prohibitively expensive.

The impossibility of tiny baby John's birth, of my brother's birth, too, opens up possibility. We struggle with birth, we contend with it, because it's the kind of impossible thing women do every day.

LaRee tells me she loves her daughter Tara. She's praying for her. She believes she'll come home. She doesn't want to talk about the book. She's writing her own book, which she will give to her grandchildren. She will not let me see this book.

Instead, we talk for two hours about birth. She shows me her Bible for homebirth: *Polly's Birth Book*, a self-published book by Polly Block. Block was a Mormon midwife, a midwife legend, LaRee tells me. Polly died in 2007, but her daughter Jeanette now sells the book through a Facebook page that asks, "What would you do if there was a natural disaster? Or hospitals were 'unavailable'?" Polly was a prepper who once buried a stove under the ground, just in case.[5]

Amazon reviews of the book and testimonials on the website all tell stories of couples using *Polly's Birth Book* to have unassisted home births. Writes one husband, "It is our hope that others will have the courage to choose homebirth, assisted or unassisted. We know that it will bless the moms, babies, and families involved, and help to mend the rampant societal disconnect that is driving so many children to gangs, drugs, and other negative behaviors."

The book is a terrifying DIY handbook. For placental abruption, a life-threatening condition when the placenta detaches prematurely from the inside of the uterus, Polly recommends 1 teaspoon of cayenne in ½ cup of cold water and "TRANSPORT TO THE HOSPITAL AS QUICKLY AS POSSIBLE." For placenta previa, another life-threatening condition when the placenta lies low in the uterus and obscures the cervix, Polly recommends, "NOTIFY A PHYSICIAN. Cold HVC (honey, vinegar, and cayenne, in water) should be taken for bleeding."[6]

I read the book as LaRee talks about all the babies she's delivered all over the county. I am incredulous. I am afraid. I am in awe. I believe her and also I don't. I wonder at the capacity of my body and its stories.

LaRee tells me one story of how she held a woman's hemorrhaging uterus inside her body while she transported her to the hospital.

We talk as men walk in and out of the large room. Shawn is one of them, Val another. LaRee tells me about miracles and birth. She speaks both words with one breath. With the next breath, they flow into betrayal and stories. When I came here, their family lawyer told me that LaRee and Val would not talk about Tara's book. But the book is all they talk about. They tell me which specific passages are untrue. Often, as they tell a story, LaRee says, "See, how could Tara be right if this story I am telling is true?" They talk about the book when they tell me about the truth about the Lord, about stories, about understanding.

The Amazon reviews of *Educated* are filled with voices of family members and friends, each vying for the truth. One of Westover's brothers, Travis, shares part of an email he sent to his sister in 2016:

> Usually in reports of scientific and engineering projects we follow what is known as the "80/20 rule," which is that reports focus on key messages and points and deliberately leave out seemingly contradictory or excessively complicated information for general audiences. The fact is that practically no-one can understand all of the details in a complicated situation, and focusing on the underlying themes is generally best unless the audience has specific need to try to grasp the details. I think that you did well following the 80/20 rule. If you like I could send clarifying notes that you could include in an appendix or as publication notes. As you mention, we have different memories and different perceptions of the same events, and I recognize that if you try to include my version, it will likely interfere with your clean narrative.[7]

I read that comment before I went out to Idaho. It reminded me of an email my own brother sent me in 2014, after I sent him thirty thousand words of a story I was working on about our family. Thirty thousand words I never finished:

> What I think your story did was capture the "spirit" of what it was like growing up in our family with 100% accuracy. Meaning, even if some of the stories in actuality may have happened in a slightly different way, that person actually said this or that, and it actually happened this way or that, it doesn't matter because in the end this is a story of you and how you were

impacted by all of these events, which imbues the story with its own "truth."

I bring in the voices of the brothers to complicate the narrative. To throw everything into doubt while reaffirming it. To challenge our origin stories while defending them. Whenever there's more than one person in a story, there's more than one story. The problem with birth is that we believe there can be only one.

In her short story "Giving Birth," Margaret Atwood writes, "But who gives it? And to whom is it given? Certainly it doesn't feel like giving, which implies a flow, a gentle handing over, no coercion. . . . No one ever says giving death, although they are in some ways the same, events, not things. And *delivering*, the act the doctor is generally believed to perform: who delivers what? Is it the mother who is delivered like a prisoner released?"[8]

I was born the day my daughter was born. I was born again with my son. I was born the day I wrote one story of my life, and I am born again every time I write another, and another. If my children write, I will be remade in their stories, but it will not remake who I am.

My mother and I no longer share our narratives with each other. I long for hers, but she, like LaRee, withholds it. These mothers both know that I will take their stories like a greedy child and spin them out and out and out, until I have made a whole life of the thing they have given me.

During our talk, LaRee told me I would lie about this trip. "I will fact-check," I told her. "I have notes and I am recording. I will reach out to confirm the details."

"I've worked with fact-checkers before—you all lie, everyone lies," she said.

I could hear her anger, and I knew it could not be appeased. "Do you want me to leave?" I asked. "I will leave. I will drive away and I will not bother you again."

But, "No," she said. "God told me you should be here, so here you are."

Later, a magazine editor I was working with on a version of this story asked to go out and take some pictures, and LaRee said she would only let the photographer come out if I let her see a draft of the story.

"I can't do that," I told her. "This story isn't about this, anyway. This story is about everything and I have to write it in a particular way, which I don't know yet, which I can't know yet until it comes out of me."

It's the silliest, most mystical thing I have ever written about a story. But it's also the most true.

I canceled the assignment with the editor.

I was in Clifton two nights and I was in the middle of so much beauty and I had never felt more trapped. The last night I was there, LaRee took me to dinner with her son Shawn and some of his children, including John. They are so wonderful, those children. So beautiful and smart. I love them. I thought about my siblings and our lives. I wrote down the names of these children, who reminded me of us, but promised never to publish them. Their story isn't for me to tell.

John came to sit with me. I told him knock-knock jokes and he told me some classics about why the chicken crossed the road.

Then, "I'm a miracle baby," he told me in a whisper. "Did you know that I am a miracle?"

And I told him I believe his story with my whole entire heart.

Part IV

FOURTH TRIMESTER

Oh, sorry, did you think you were done? Did you think this was over? Did you think that once you had that baby, that was it? No, no, and no. Welcome to the fourth trimester. The three months it takes for your baby to adjust outside of the womb and for you to adjust to them.

Your baby is no longer a fruit or vegetable. Your baby is a person. Your baby is crying. Your baby is pooping. Your baby is driving you crazy. You love your baby, but your vagina is still bleeding and that first postpartum poop made you cry. You love your baby, but you've forgotten how to shower. You love your baby, but your nipples are raw and you bled on your baby's nose, dropped guacamole on his head when you desperately tried to eat while you fed him. You're famished. Your body looks like a deflated balloon. Don't even bother looking at the raw meat of your swollen vulva or the tender line of your C-section scar. The heaving boulders of your breasts.

Your shoe size might be different. Your hair might be curlier. Or maybe it's straight now. Or a different color. Did you know these things could happen? Did you know the chemical makeup of who and what you are has changed, forever?

Did you know your baby is crying?

Congratulations, you are a night walker. You are a night crier. You dwell in the caverns of time when everyone else seems to be sleeping or working. You live in moments that you didn't know existed. In a world full of crying (from both you and the baby) and leaking urine (from both you and the baby).

You will walk differently while holding your baby, imagining all the ways you can fall, all the horrible accidents that could happen. You will fear tripping while you hold the baby, slipping, being bumped, or doing the bumping. The images running through your mind are like scenes from the movie *Final Destination*—there are so many ways to die. Now that you have given life, death haunts you. Is the baby still breathing? You will check and recheck. Is the baby sleeping too long? Did the baby not sleep long enough? Did the baby cry too much? Why isn't my baby crying?

One day you will sleep. But not now.

Congratulations, did you know your baby is crying, again?

If you are lucky, you can stay home. But LOL if you think you are getting anything done. LOL if you think you are going to clean or take up knitting. Instead, you will exist in this new world, the baby's world. Your existence will consist of three stages: feeding, sleeping, and cleaning up poop. You will slip through them, back and forth and back and forth. It is endless. But it will end, so make sure you enjoy it.

If you are not lucky, you are working again. You are wearing uncomfortable clothes—nothing fits—tight against your still-tender body, answering email or calls, picking up a broom or stacking boxes. Our society doesn't allow you to recover. You aren't supposed to.

If you are lucky, your office has a room where you can pump. Or an office door you can close. Maybe you have to ask for this and go through the awkward insistence on your legal rights, while people sigh heavily and offer you a conference room or a closet. Or maybe you don't even ask because you just know you can't win and who can afford a breast pump anyway? And who can afford the time it takes? And who can juggle the bottles of milk and their refrigeration needs along with a job and children and the whole weight of life crushing on you?

Your body is supposed to bounce back. You are supposed to find that pre-baby body, ASAP. But it's like the lost city of Atlantis. Don't even argue with me here. Don't. If you tell me you've found it, I have to assume you're lying, probably to sell me an expensive smoothie, or essential oils, or laxative teas. Stop it immediately. After all, your baby is still crying. They need you.

Ice Diapers

Five years after giving birth for the last time, I cleaned out my freezer in preparation to leave my marriage. Every big moment in my adult life I have marked by cleaning my freezer. It's a subconscious ritual. Publish a book? Clean the freezer. End a twelve-year marriage? Clean the freezer.

At the back of the freezer, I found a diaper. It was what the nurses had called an ice diaper. They showed me how to make ice diapers at the hospital after the birth of my first child. You take a disposable baby diaper and run it under water. Freeze it flat. They make handy ice packs for the bleeding, swollen mess of your vulva.

Ice diapers and mesh hospital underwear were the two things I did not know I would love until suddenly I did. Until I survived sixteen hours of labor and four hours of pushing and a few minutes of my doctor using the handheld vacuum apparatus to get that baby the fuck out of my vaginal canal, and my lower half felt like a Vegas hotel room after it had been trashed by a B-list rock band.

After giving birth, the first time I stood up to go to the bathroom I peed myself. The urine just poured out of me like my bladder was a cup tipped over. I stared at the nurse, horrified.

"Aren't I supposed to feel something there? Shouldn't I have felt that coming?"

She shrugged. "It happens." They mopped it up.

The soft brush of the forgiving hospital mesh underwear slipping over my ass was the only caress I wanted after giving birth. No one could touch me, only my kid and the mesh underwear and ice diapers. I recoiled from hugs. My skin vibrated with exhaustion. The kind of tired I could feel in my eye sockets.

Everything was different. I couldn't shower without strapping the baby into the Rock 'N Play in the bathroom with me and turning on white noise—theoretically so I could soothe her, but in reality all it did was drown out her cries long enough for me to shampoo my hair and wash spit-up off my skin. I soon learned not to shower. Cleanliness, like resistance, was futile.

I had entered the postnatal period called the fourth trimester. The term "fourth trimester" is attributed to Harvey Karp in his 2002 book *The Happiest Baby on the Block*. Karp defines it as the baby's first three months of life, when you and the baby are adjusting to them living outside the womb.

The American Academy of Pediatrics recommends that infants receive their first well-child check three to five days after birth and then again at 1, 2, 4, 6, 9, 12, 15, 18, and 24 months. Mothers who had a vaginal delivery are given just one postpartum checkup at six weeks.

Just one.

That's it.

Is it any surprise, then, that infant mortality rates are declining in the United States even as maternal mortality rates—which account for women who die during pregnancy, childbirth, or the crucial first forty-two days postdelivery—are rising?[1]

During the fourth trimester, postpartum parents are still bleeding from a vaginal birth or recovering from a C-section. Since

1952, the United Nations International Labor Organization has called for a minimum of fourteen weeks of paid maternity leave for all employed women. In some nations, like Cuba and Mongolia, mothers are entitled to twelve months of paid leave. Other countries, like Norway, Sweden, and Canada, offer six months of paid leave. Russia guarantees women about four and a half months of paid leave at 100 percent of their salary. All of these programs are government funded.

The United States is one of only eight countries in the United Nations that doesn't guarantee paid leave. And five of those countries are small Pacific islands. The United States is one of the wealthiest nations in the world, but we are among the most tight-fisted when it comes to helping mothers. One in four US mothers returns to work within two months of giving birth, and one in ten go back after only four weeks.[2] This lack of access to paid leave particularly impacts low-income workers and women of color, who experience higher maternal mortality rates.[3]

One of the theories for why the United States lags behind European countries in paid leave is that, after World War II, European countries needed to encourage women to enter the workforce to rebuild cities and national economies. The United States, which had profited from a robust wartime economy, incurred fewer casualties, and suffered little damage, needed women to leave the workforce.[4]

Paid or even unpaid protected leave seemed like a pipe dream. Up until 1978, when the Pregnancy Discrimination Act (PDA) amended the 1964 Civil Rights Act, pregnant women and mothers in the United States could legally be fired—or not hired in the first place—just for being pregnant or having children. Of course, to this day there are employers who break the law and employees who can't bear the potential cost or reputational backlash of trying to hold them accountable.

Since that battle was won (mostly), progress has been incremental. The next front was the push for family leave. One of the earliest iterations of the Family and Medical Leave Act, proposed in 1984, called for twenty-six weeks of unpaid leave for parenting a new child or for caring for an ill child or spouse. The bill was amended and merged with other proposals and debated for years, and when it was finally passed in 1990, President George H. W. Bush vetoed it.

Bill Clinton would sign the FMLA in 1993. But by that point it had been so watered down that it only provided for twelve weeks of unpaid time off—less than half of what the original had called for. And it applies only to private sector employees who have worked for their employer for at least twelve months. Private sector employers who employ fewer than fifty employees are not subject to FMLA.

More recently, in 2013, Senator Kirsten Gillibrand (D-NY) pushed for a bill that would guarantee sixty days of paid maternity leave at 66 percent of a worker's wages (capped at $1,000 a week) and establish an office of paid family and medical leave inside the Social Security Administration. That bill was sent to committee in 2015 and hasn't been seen again.[5]

Then, the 2016 election ushered in a new administration, with its own ideas and priorities. Under the Trump administration, Ivanka Trump promised to push for paid family leave even as she denied it to workers at her own fashion company. Her policy, announced in 2019, proposed a solution where parents could pull from Social Security for paid family leave—a plan that would serve only to compound inequality: wealthier workers who could save for retirement would be able to draw on their benefits without worrying, while low-income workers would have to put off retirement.

This isn't just about the health of the postpartum parent, although that ought to be enough. But, as we know, it all too often isn't. Just as the life of a hypothetical human is prioritized over the welfare of the fully embodied flesh-and-blood adult carrying them in their womb, we prioritize caring for the new baby over offering any support to the new parent, who is bleeding while sitting on an ice diaper begging someone, anyone, to just let them sleep. Even though they might also be able to offer better care for the baby if they were given access to better support for themselves.

A European study published in 2000 found that forty weeks of paid leave decreased the rate of infant death by 20 percent.[6] Paid leave also correlates with a decline in postpartum depression.[7] Other studies back this up. Taking care of parents saves the lives of infants. But our government isn't acting to do so, and neither are our nation's doctors.

The World Health Organization recommends four postnatal care visits to a doctor for a mother in the first six weeks.[8] The American College of Obstetricians and Gynecologists simply recommends insurance reimbursement for an individualized plan for postpartum care.[9] But what does that even mean? It's up to insurance plans to decide. So, it's a wholly inadequate recommendation that gives the care of our bodies over to the companies that profit off of us.

In the 2018 movie *Tully*, Charlize Theron plays Marlo, a mother of two who's pregnant with an unplanned third. Her son has an undiagnosed developmental disorder, which puts Marlo at odds with his school and makes her the target of his frustrated rages.

Exhausted after the birth of her third child, Marlo shuffles through her life, with circles under her eyes, draped in a stretched-out cardigan. She moves from one feeding to another to another. Diaper change. Feeding. Time passes, but it doesn't seem to. The movie shows this as a montage of dull and painful and exhausted repetitions—changing diapers, waking up, nursing. Repeat. Marlo is stuck in a world without help, without resources, chained to the care of her children. She's lucky, though, because she doesn't have to work.

I saw the movie not long after I left my marriage. Sitting in an empty theater, with popcorn and wine, I was without my children, who for so long had defined my existence.

In 2013, after the birth of my son, with the cost of nonsubsidized childcare eating up the low wages I received as a writer, I had quit my job and become a stay-at-home mom. I balanced freelance work with coupon cutting and budgeting so we could make ends meet on one salary. My husband complained about the money I spent on food and clothes, because the cost of children was more than he expected, but when I eagerly offered to find a full-time job, he complained about the cost of day care. So, I would work at night or early in the morning, then take care of the children, who were just over two years apart. There was a low-cost preschool that took my toddler for sixteen hours each week, but I still had an infant to care for. And then there was grocery shopping and house cleaning and cooking. Whenever I tried to ask for help with these tasks, my husband complained or, worse, asked me to make him a chore chart.

The chore chart broke me. I wouldn't do it. "You are not a thirteen-year-old," I told him.

Only twice did I see him vacuum. One of those times was when I was recovering from a kidney infection that had landed me in the emergency room.

When my son was a newborn, screaming nonstop between the hours of four p.m. and seven p.m., I begged my husband to bring home food—McDonald's hamburgers, anything—just to take some work off my plate.

He never did.

I remember holding my wailing son, walking him through the house, while my toddler daughter watched a TV show, waiting for my husband to come home. I would press my face to the window and imagine myself setting my son on the floor, opening the door, and running away. I would run down the street, barefoot, and disappear. My imagination only took me as far as the point where I vanished, like a ghost, from my life. After that, there was no plan. Just run.

Every week, I would clean my desperate nose prints off the windowpane. Every week, they would reappear.

Watching *Tully*, seeing that montage, I began to sob.

The exhaustion breaks Marlo. She decides to take her brother up on the offer of a night nurse. A generous offer she had previously refused. The night nurse, Tully, allows Marlo to sleep, allows her to rest, allows her to become more vibrant. The women even have a threesome with Marlo's husband. Everything is perfect, until Tully tells Marlo she has to go.

That night, Marlo crashes her car into a lake after falling asleep at the wheel. When she wakes up, she learns that Tully was a fiction her exhausted brain invented. Everything that Tully did was Marlo doing it all along. At the end of the movie, we see Marlo shuffling through her life once again, only this time, her husband is at her side.

That was the moment in the movie I stopped crying. Instead, I got irritated. It had been nice to see my life reflected on the screen for a small moment, but the ease with which the story wrangles out of answering its questions felt cheap. It had taken a near-death experience on the part of this man's wife for him to do some baseline labor for his family? Was I supposed to find him sympathetic? Was this supposed to be kindness? Was this supposed to be hope?

The truth is, it does take hitting rock bottom for people to notice we're drowning. The movie is small and intimate and finely wrought, but not radical. This dark underbelly of motherhood is everywhere, we just refuse to see it until we are forced to.

My favorite genre of internet essay is the "No one ever told me" genre, in which women who seemingly haven't picked up a contemporary novel written by a mother in the last hundred years complain that no one ever told them motherhood would be hard.

When my friend Mel said this to her own mother, just days after bringing her first child home from the hospital, her mother laughed. "Oh, honey, we told you, you just didn't listen."

Amy Nelson, the founder of the coworking space for women called The Riveter, is pushing for corporate change. Her Instagram story is full of images of her three daughters and bags of her breastmilk. We see her getting up early to work out with her postpartum body and all glammed up, holding her baby at a meeting. Another female founder of a women's coworking space, Audrey Gelman of The Wing, was pictured pregnant on the cover of *Inc.* magazine. The image was heralded by Parade.com as "Awesome AF." Noted in the article is that employers are biased against mothers in the workplace, who are seen as less capable and less dedicated.[10]

These women are working to change corporate culture's ideas about working mothers. But the face of this new vision for businesswomen who don't have to hide their kids to be taken seriously is still limited to attractive white women. (A fact these CEOs would concede.) And all this exposure is still leaving women out in the cold. All of this polished performance art of our bodies and our milk and our blood.

What does it all mean without legislation? Without policies and laws to back it up? The visibility of smiling rich white mothers and their problems generally helps only smiling rich white mothers.

We know the problems that face new mothers. We've written books and books and books about them. But for all our glossy representation, we've failed to change the system. Women are instead told *they* need to change—to "lean in" or "wash their faces" as Sheryl Sandberg's and Rachel Hollis's best-selling books, respectively, dictate. But it's a solution that dodges fundamental and structural change.

By making the solution individual, something women should do for themselves, we give women yet another job. "I have identified the problem," neoliberalism says, "and it's on you to fix"—by working harder or hiring a housecleaner or using an app to help you accomplish tasks. Each prescription insidiously papers over the problem rather than solving it. And so the most privileged people pay—and "lean in"—their way around deep structural inequities, while those most in need are given one more task to feel like they're failing at.

Writing in *New York Magazine*'s The Cut, Jen Gann sounds just as exhausted as the rest of us when she asks, after watching *Tully*, "Just how many gnarly depictions of motherhood are necessary for anything to change? If our laws and policies reflected the challenges of parenthood, perhaps we wouldn't feel such pangs upon seeing a counter soaked in breast milk. In the theater where I watched *Tully*, when Marlo's Medela bag toppled, women gasped into the darkness."[11]

I'll add a caveat to Gann's analysis: we may be so saturated with representations of overwhelmed white, straight, cisgender, middle- and upper-class, able-bodied mothers that seeing another can feel like trauma porn, but meanwhile mothers and trans and nonbinary parents who don't fit within that narrowly defined range of acceptable characteristics often don't have the same freedom to show they're struggling. The label "bad mother" is used too freely and always carries a sting. But it's more bark than bite for people who look like our culture's maternal ideal, those who don't have to work twice as hard to be seen as a good parent. For others, if they don't succeed, they risk social alienation, having child services called on them, and being seen as confirming vicious stereotypes about their race, sexuality, gender identity, class, or disability. If we did listen to their stories with the same compassion and empathy we reserve for relatively privileged mothers, what then? We might have to actually come to terms with the reality that our culture around motherhood is in dire need of an overhaul, and no amount of "personal responsibility" can save us.

Postpartum care in America is fucked, and so are parental leave policies. And these inequalities disproportionately affect parents who are low-income or minorities. The solutions of storytelling and greater visibility only seem to raise the profile of well-off white women.

What's next? Is this where I offer policy solutions? Or tell you to keep your chin up, mama? Or maybe I post a picture of me with my cellulite, backlit so I look good when it goes viral?

Or, instead, is this where I tell us to stop making viral videos about how hard it all is and to start lobbying Congress to pass some parental leave because our nation is working hard to overturn *Roe v. Wade* in the name of saving babies but won't let moms get a goddamn night's sleep? So many other women have made this argument and we didn't listen. Way back in 1989, in sociologist Arlie Russell Hochschild's groundbreaking book *The Second Shift*, she declared the fight to give women equal opportunities in the workplace and get their male partners to take up an equal share of the responsibilities in the home a stalled revolution.[12] Hochschild is a professor emeritus at Berkeley and won a

Guggenheim! But no one seemed to listen to her. So you sure as hell won't listen to me.

What will it take to convince Americans to change the status quo? We're already dying, while our politicians pass medically and constitutionally unsound laws to save the babies. How many deaths and thwarted lives, how much pain and suffering will it take to make us care? Will we ever? Or will we continually find ways for certain people to waltz around the gaping potholes of our social infrastructure, choosing capitalism over structural change?

Cleaning out the freezer, before I moved out of our house, I grabbed the ice diaper. I thought about shoving it in my pants, sitting on it. Would it feel good? The idea seemed silly. Whatever relief it had provided to my throbbing, bleeding vulva had been temporary. And whatever it offered me now was only a reminder of what I'd had to overcome, myself.

I put the ice diaper in the trash.

Mom Bod

To go for a run, I had to wake up before five in the morning or face peeling tiny hands off of my thighs later.

"Mommy will only be gone for an hour," I would tell them, in a voice that I hoped didn't convey my irritation. Their hands are so small; they pull and grab. The baby likes to stand on my feet, clutch my leg, and wail wet-faced into my thigh. My daughter jerks my arms, paws my calves, turns her face into my crotch and cries. Her *please don't go!* vibrates my skin and I push her aside. I want to be gentle, I want to be kind, but I also need to be free.

My husband leans in for a kiss. His hands brush my shoulders. I smell his breath; I can feel the promise of whiskers scratch my lips. Their love is overwhelming; I want to shove it all away.

I escape and shut the door behind me. I know they are confused. I can see my husband's look, the one that says "I just wanted to kiss you. Why don't you kiss me back?" in a single glance. It's bemused, a little irritated, grudgingly resigned. And even through the window of the door, my children are reaching for me, their wet lips, clawing hands press against the panes. I am running away from their insistent claims of manifest destiny on my body.

My whole life people have had plans for my body. Men have wanted to fuck it. Pastors have wanted to preserve it. My parents wanted to control it, to shield me from its complicated desires and needs. My children use it to feed—first their bodies and then their hearts. This is why I run, to remember what it is like to have my body belong to me alone. The pain in my side, the ache in my knees: These are mine. Inflicted by me. They are my choice.

But even on runs, I can still feel the weight of others' plans for me. The hot-breathed honking. I give them the finger; they drive away. When I give the finger on my runs, I am putting down a flag, staking a claim, saying: I own this. This isn't for you. What you see ambling and sweating up that hill is not yours, buddy. Not today. Not ever.

Every gaze carries an expectation for my flesh. I am supposed to be demure and modest. I'm supposed to be fit. We don't celebrate the sex appeal of "mom bods." I'm supposed to be a hot mom. A healthy mom. I'm supposed to nourish with this body, lift weights with this body, pound cement with the heavy heels of this body. I'm supposed to make love with this body. Wake up at night and soothe with this body. I'm supposed to cinch this body. Spanx this body. Bra this body. Firm this body. Soften my body. Make up my body. Peel and wax and buff my body. Everywhere I see exhortations: to embrace my body, love my body, heal my body, nurture my body, tone my body, slim my body.

Sometimes I forget that it is, in fact, my body.

When my children were born, I was dedicated to breastfeeding them. Pamphlets, websites, books, and my doctor had all convinced me that breastfeeding was the right call—truly the only call—to make as a mother. The American Academy of Pediatrics recommends that infants be exclusively breastfed for about the first six months, a year if possible. Breastfed babies are supposed to be smarter and happier and more well-adjusted. In my prenatal class, the lactation consultant had us all give our mothers (none of whom were in the room) a round of applause for breastfeeding us. I wanted to breastfeed. I did.

My breasts, which swelled from A cups to Es, seemed to want to as well. But we couldn't figure it out. My squirming, starving daughter struggled to get a latch. My swollen breasts got clogged, so I pumped and pumped, building up a huge stash. She got so little breastmilk from the actual source, I began to give her bottles. She sucked these bottles dry. Soon, I was pumping exclusively and giving her bottle after bottle. She bulked up into a fat and happy baby and our system of pumping and bottle feeding worked because I worked only part-time and I had only one child.

But I hated it. It took me forty-five minutes to pump. Sitting there, listening to the mechanical *wah-wah-wah-wah*, I felt like a cow. Worse than a cow—their milking machines are much more effective.

When my daughter was nine months old, I got the flu and quit pumping. I was throwing up, exhausted, and just didn't care. She was a happy, fat baby. My stash at home depleted, and I began cutting the milk with formula. She didn't know the difference.

When I had my son, the idea of pumping again filled me with fear. I couldn't do it; I couldn't sit there for hours and hours hooked up to that machine. He would either breastfeed or he'd get formula, I told my husband, who balked at this plan. We fought. I told him he didn't get a choice because it was my body. He said he did because it was his child.

His disapproval and my stubborn refusal had us at an impasse. I couldn't pump. When the nurse brought my new breast pump to the hospital room after my son's birth, I had a panic attack, sobbing and sweating. At home, I locked it in the attic and then donated it to a women's shelter six months later without ever taking it out of the box. But breastfeeding was difficult this time around, too. My nipples bled. Pain shot through the tender muscles of my chest.

I asked the lactation consultant to my home to watch me feed him. "I am not doing this right," I told her. "I don't feel right. My body hurts so much."

She glanced at me and shrugged. "You'll figure it out."

Three hours later, my mom arrived for a visit and saw me crying on the floor. I was sweating and my chest burned with pain.

She, who had nursed seven children and pumped for her eighth, took one look and sent me to the doctor. I had mastitis. If the lactation consultant had really seen me, really listened, she would have sent me to the doctor as well.

After that, nursing went better with my son. It had to; he refused to take a bottle. Now, instead of being chained to a machine, I was chained to my child.

In my small moments away, when I would try to escape to the grocery store, inevitably my husband would call, with the baby screaming in the background. "You need to come home," he'd tell me. Once I answered the phone and all I heard was the baby screaming. And then he hung up.

I quit breastfeeding when my son was nine months old. I couldn't handle it. With every new stage in his development, every change in his latch, my nipples would bleed and scab over. I found a bottle that the baby would take, and then I left for a weekend visit to a friend in another state. When I came back, he had moved to the bottle.

In her book *Lactivism*, Courtney Jung argues that our society often promotes the benefits of breastfeeding to the detriment of mothers. We share exaggerated claims of the benefits of breastfeeding, causing postpartum parents who can't breastfeed, for either medical or personal reasons, to spiral into guilt. The reality, Jung points out, is that the science on the extent of breastfeeding's benefits is inconclusive. Many studies on breastfeeding are observational rather than randomized controlled trials. The women who are most likely to breastfeed are those who have the time to breastfeed, meaning they trend wealthier and white. So, what look like the benefits of breastfeeding in a child could just be the benefits of having parents with the money to buy time.[1] Of course we know there are proven benefits to breastfeeding, but there are also costs. The literature and culture around breastfeeding are less about outcomes and more about control. The relentless push to force women to breastfeed reinforces the narrative that the mother's body exists for the sole purpose of growing the child, even now. A vessel once again.

As usual, it's a trap. Women are told to breastfeed and then shamed for breastfeeding in public. It's yet another manifestation of the constant cultural tension between telling a woman what her body is made to be used for, while also telling her to put it away because it's disgusting or sexual and no one wants to see it.

In a genre of viral mom content I like to call "defiant breastfeeding mom," a recent winner is a picture of a mother breastfeeding her infant with the breastfeeding cover draped over her own head instead of the baby's. The caption reads: "A friend's daughter-in-law was told to 'cover up' while feeding her baby, so she did! I've never met her, but I think she's AWESOME!!! (Please share! With permission, I've made this post public—I'm SO over people shaming women for nursing!!!)"

Every year, women go viral with this sort of content. It's relatable. Any woman who has tried to nurse has experienced the side-eye of a judgy woman or uncomfortable man. When I was breastfeeding my son, my brother-in-law saw me nursing in the living room of his mom's house. "Are you going to do that here?" he asked.

"Are *you* gonna be a jerk to me here?" I asked.

He left the room.

If this were about science, studies that show that babies who are formula-fed are just fine and healthy would be part of the narrative, right alongside the studies about the benefits of breastfeeding. We'd present women with the information and then support them with their choice—because it *is* their choice. At least, it should be. But somehow it's not, and it never has been. Whether the alternative is wet nurses or formula, women have always been told there is a right choice and a wrong choice. Which is which has waxed and waned with each new cultural understanding of what a woman—and by extension, what a mother—should be. Jacqueline Wolf explains in her book *Don't Kill Your Baby* that breastfeeding rates in America dropped as women went to work during the Industrial Revolution. But they rose again when backlash against women in the workplace sent them home again. The same drop in breastfeeding rates seen during World War II rose again in the postwar era. The La Leche League was founded in 1956, and between that and the rise of the natural birth movement in the 1970s, breastfeeding continued to gain in popularity.[2]

The expectations change constantly. Women can't seem to win. We aren't supposed to win. The game is rigged. Your job is to try to meet an impossible standard, and you will always fail, and your failure will drive you to try harder and harder, never once lifting your head to see how fucked the system is. Never once questioning what it is you want, who you are, or what your body is meant to do.

After graduating college, before children, I got married and started running races. My father-in-law asked me to run a half marathon with him. So I trained, moaning against the slow monotony of my tread, the pain in my arch from my flat feet, my swollen ankles.

My father-in-law pushed me. He had run full marathons. He loved to talk about how his skin bled during his first marathon. How he ran one with a bee sting swelling his arm.

As I ran, I learned to inhabit my body more fully. The me inside grew to fill up this awkward flesh I'd been given. I learned its grooves, its hidden places, and its needs. I was learning similar lessons in my new marriage. We had been virgins, but he didn't own me in the way I had been told he would. Instead, we learned each other and learned ourselves. I was lucky; he only wanted what I was willing to give. And I gave only what I knew, and what I knew we learned together—a syllabus of hesitancy, tenderness, and awkwardness at night. And pain and plodding and pushing during the day.

The month before I was to run the half, my father-in-law called. He insisted both my husband and I be on the phone. So, we picked up both handsets (it was a landline then) and stood side by side in the same room.

"I have cancer," I heard my father-in-law say.

That's all I remember. I know I stood there. I know I listened. But all that registered was the pain seeping over the phone, pulling us into a riptide of fear.

The cancer was advanced. We never got to run the race together. He wanted to, but his sons didn't want him to. His wife didn't want him to. He could barely walk. "I can walk and cheer you on," he said, when I told him it wasn't a good idea.

"But your immune system," my brother-in-law reminded him.

"I won't run it. I'm not doing that to you," I said. I was afraid of being his last trip, his last outing, and his last choice. I didn't want him to do it for me.

So, we didn't run together. We didn't run it at all. Years later, I would understand how much he wanted to have that last race and how we had all conspired to rob him of it. I see it now as his assertion of self. Already the chemo had begun. Already he was ceding control of his body to doctors and family. But this would have been his choice—to, one last time, propel his body through the air, for no other reason than to feel his own legs move beneath him.

He died eight months later. Killed by an uprising in his own cells. When he went into hospice, his abdomen was distended with medicine and fluids and his mind was no longer lucid. He kept insisting that he needed to run. That someone should bring him his shoes so he could run.

I know now that this is common for patients in hospice. The almost-dead are always trying to flee. Death is a process of slowly ceding yourself, so it makes sense that they just want that one last race, to once more feel their legs thrust them forward, to stake their claim to their own bodies and wills.

I ran the half the next year. I was so slow that the full-marathon runners were passing me by the time I made it to mile twelve. When I crossed the finish line, I wanted to cry but couldn't—I didn't have anything left in me. I felt wrung out and spent and deliriously happy with my own body and all I'd required of it. It's cliché, but I had never felt so alive.

Just when I felt my body had become mine, I had a child. Pregnancy caused my body to turn on me, to become a stranger. I grew a small tumor, caused by pregnancy hormones, that bled down my back. I couldn't stop the nausea. I couldn't stop the weight gain. All I could do was watch myself grow. Other people came to stake their claims. The women who touched my stomach, the men who told me I must be due any day now. Once I bought California rolls from a restaurant and the cashier looked at me and said, "I thought pregnant women weren't supposed to have sushi."

I took my receipt and gave her the finger.

I didn't know how to walk. I didn't know how to move. I was completely possessed by another human in a way that felt both deeply magical and sinister.

Who am I? I asked after my daughter was born. My body—now size 16, with size E breasts—took up space differently, moved through the world differently. My stippled flesh hung loose and raw. It took sixteen hours of labor, four hours of pushing, before she'd been hoovered from me with a hand-pump vacuum. It seemed so primitive, and so necessary.

"Whatever," I said, when the doctor asked if it was okay to bring out the vacuum. "I'm done. Just get it out." With my last push, I fainted. When I opened my eyes, they'd placed her on me—red skin, mucus, blood, and a web of vernix. Completely me, completely her own. Again, I wanted to cry. Again, I was too spent. Everything I could produce I already had, and here she was, lying on me, her blue eyes wide.

Two years later, another baby. Again my body waxed and waned. Pregnancy is an intensely physical pursuit. We stretch wide, we swell, we push, we bleed. We are torn, stitched, put back together.

After both births, I started running again as soon as possible. Putting two sports bras on my giant boobs, double bagging them. Squeezing into my running shorts and shirts, which would fit again one day, but didn't yet.

Every run takes me away, but it also brings me back to those little bodies that need mine. The bodies just learning to separate their need from my skin, their love from my arms—I push against the pain, but gentler now than I did before. I know how to settle in. I know how to push my shoulders back and straighten my spine. I know how to find my stride and fill my lungs. I know how to inhabit this body, my body.

I understand my father-in-law better now.

As I think about the body I inhabit and how it has widened and narrowed and widened again, and how I've struggled within its limits, I often think of a 2009 interview, in which Mary Gaitskill notes, "We come into these physical bodies . . . whatever we are takes this shape that is so particular and distinct—eyes, nose, mouth—and then it gradually begins to disintegrate. Eventually it's going to dissolve completely."[3]

What a strange life, to be placed in flesh and told that it is you. To be told that you are what you see in the mirror. And then before you can get comfortable in it, the world lays claim to it. Your body must. Your body should.

When I hear these claims, I lace up my running shoes. My body is still slow. I have no desire to be fast, I no longer need to bleed or bruise. All I want to do is fill up what's inside. To connect to the skin. To navigate the space I am required to take up in the world. This is me and this isn't me. I understand now why in their last days the dying want to run. They want to run away from the thing that is holding them back and dissolve into themselves again. So do I.

Context

The flight attendant lost her wings. They pinged on the ground as she walked by checking the cabin before our flight. They were brass and felt heavy in my hands. The pin was bent and it pricked my palm as I hid them in my lap. I wanted to steal them. I am thirty-two, the mother of two children. But that was in my normal life. In that moment on the airplane, I was on an escape, flying from Chicago to Portland, where I would be attending a weeklong writing workshop. The trip was a chance to slough off the skin of mother and wife for a week and just be a writer. To just be me.

I had no business stealing the wing pin. I didn't really want it. But as the plane took off and we hovered over the land, I wanted to be—just for a moment—the kind of person who might.

When people see me, they see a mother. I do my best, but the signs are all there: diapers spilling from my purse, Cheerios falling from my wallet, a Dora sticker on my ass. Most of my days are spent in the company of two small children, who demand cheese sticks and games of hide and seek and who always seem to have some remnant of a meal they barely ate stuck to their cheeks. Each moment is a small drama, with a narrative arc that seems to capture all of life's greatest struggles. "My Brother Wants My Fairy Wings" is a story of howling desire, of capitalism, of pain and sibling rivalry. And it all takes place in two yowling minutes before the "My Sister Is Taking Up All the Room in the Whole House and Needs to Stop Breathing on Me" melodrama commences.

I write in moments that feel like I'm plunging underwater. During naptime, while the baby sings himself to sleep and my daughter plays with her toys. Before she demands a computer game or the baby wakes up yelling for waffles. In the mornings, after my run, my thighs stick to the office chair as I type out a sentence or two, before I hear yet another holler for waffles. Or at night, after their bedtime, while I listen to my daughter sing herself a song, the chorus of which declares "When I am a mommy, I will neber put my kids in timeout for pushing each other!"

I hand off the iPad to my four-year-old so I can sneak in a few moments of writing, until the guilt consumes me and I return to her. I boomerang between what feels like polar opposite directions on the compass of my life—writing and mothering.

Before I was a mother, I was a writer. And later, when my children only need me in fits and starts, I will still be a writer. Before I wrote about them, I wrote about books and politics and sex. Now, I tell people I exploit my uterus. It's a joke, but it isn't.

I used to write listening to classical music. Now, when there is silence, I sink into it. I stretch my fingers out and feel the quiet, like it's the hem of an expensive dress I'll never buy because someone will smear it with Cheetos.

For now, writing my children is writing my body. It's hard to know where one ends and the other begins. But I feel them pulling away. I feel my writing pulling away.

I had told my husband that trip would be "a chance to really focus on my writing, you know? Without someone interrupting me to say that lions are coming out of the wall again."

I sat on the plane holding the wings. I wanted to steal them precisely because I knew that, in my normal life, I would never steal them. I wanted to steal them because, in that moment, out of context, I wanted to believe anything was possible. That I was capable of anything. That I was more than just the smear of oatmeal on my thigh.

I looked up and saw a mother with a boy my son's age: two. She was coaxing him to be still. Holding an iPad and a sucker, she cooed in his ear, words that I'm sure were "Be still and be good and you can have a treat." I know them intimately.

The boy screamed and kicked the iPad. He jumped from her lap and ran up the aisle. I put my arm out and caught him. He was bewildered. Then his little hands turned into sticky fists. I could feel the rage coming. To stave it off, I held out a pen and fished some paper from my purse. "Here, want to color?"

He grabbed them and ran back to his mother. She thanked me and I found myself explaining to her that I, too, had a boy that age. A boy who liked to kick and run and scale the cabinets. How we had to hide pie and cookies in the freezer. How he ripped a cupboard door open when the baby lock tried to stop him.

The next time the flight attendant came by, I handed her the wings.

I wasn't that person.

I have no home. The question "Where are you from?" fills me with existential dread. I am from California, Texas, South Dakota, Minnesota, Iowa. My transient childhood means that the innocuous small talk fills me with insecurity and longing. Most of the time I just say Iowa. After all, this is the place I am now. I

came here with my husband in 2005. He had a job building airplanes in Cedar Rapids and I had no other competing offers and
vague notions of graduate school.

I have lived in Iowa fourteen years now. Up until 2017, I lived
in a house where I had lived longer than in any other. The house
is ninety years old. My husband and I wrestled with the plumbing
and fought over drywall. The stairs made me bleed. I sobbed over
the state of the crown molding after we replastered the dining
room. My water broke all over the oak floors. I miscarried in the
basement bathroom, where the walls are black because the previous owners let their children develop film there.

"They were such good photographers. No one knew how to
capture a field like my son," Pat, the previous owner, told me
once. I thought of the fields reproduced in the bathroom, fields
in a land of fields, while I bled into a toilet, crushing the spiders
scurrying across the cement floor and trying not to cry.

I want to say that this is my context. The wide brushstrokes of
sky. Fields upon fields. Blankets of humidity and cold that cuts
to the bone. I want to connect myself to a land. To find a stable
foundation. Between my body and the world, I want to choose
the world. This world—the world of fields quilted together by
windbreaks of trees. The place where my children were born.
The sorrel dirt that fills their fingernails. Where I can lie between rows of corn and watch them pillar the sky.

But I can never leave my body long enough to take root. I am
always being corralled back into my skin. On a drive to a friend's
house that brought me out of town and through the countryside,
where the shadow green of soy blurred into silent waves, I heard a
horn and a boy's catcall.

"Hey, sexy mama!"

Before the truck had passed me, I was inside myself again—
pushed back from the landscape into myself. I didn't belong. Not
there. In a country of primary colors—green, blue, and red.

The landscape of the woman is the body. I am not sure I can belong anywhere else.

On the airplane, I want to escape, but I can't. The skin beneath my belly button sags. I want to offer a tissue to the teen girl next to me, who keeps wiping her nose on her sleeve. All around me there is need—the man across the aisle with yogurt in his beard, the woman with the patina of red hair and skin like discarded paper, the man with a heavy yawn, the bored girl with bright beads in her hair, that naughty little boy with hair that's only distinguishable from his skin by its gleam, teeth noticeable only because of the wide pink gaps in between, as he smiles and again kicks and again runs. And his mother—still for a moment, before reaching again to grab him. My son also has gaps like that between his teeth. I wonder if it gives him the power to kick over a chair in rage or scale the cabinets and eat piece after piece of pie until I find him, blueberry-stained lips, his cheeks filled with food and mischief.

But I have a Princess sticker stuck to the bottom of my shoe. The dress I am wearing was chosen by my four-year-old, who heard me tell my husband I was nervous to leave. She came tramping down the stairs dragging a black-and-white knit dress and a necklace. "Being fancy will help you be brave," she told me. So, I changed.

I return the boy to his mom. This is who we are, stuck in our same bodies even as we fly through the air.

I am wholly encompassed by my context—heart, thighs, bladder, hair, earlobes, sweat, the way my toes swell in their shoes, my newfound intolerance for *Law and Order: SVU*. I think about the mothers who leave. The ones who disappear and are found years later in Arizona, working as yoga instructors for retirees. I wonder how disappointed they were every night when they saw their stretch marks or peed themselves a little when they sneezed.

The reason I believe in ghosts is because if you scream loudly enough, long enough, the walls remember. We know that trauma can imprint on our DNA, so why not our walls, why not our bones? Why can't our knees forever feel the memory of our every supplication, grinding, rising up, stretching out, laying down?

I know I have been so much more than a mother. But I also know that I will never move beyond being a mother. These bodily things—spit-up and stickers, boogers and waffles—are my landscape. I will write beyond this, I will write through it and out of it. Out of my torn nails, my weak pelvic floor, the burn of my lips as I suck them in to bite between my teeth. This is the body I write in, my body.

A few days later, after I got off the plane and sequestered myself for my week of writing, I found myself hovering over a pile of books in the campus bookstore. The books were authored by the people who were teaching that week at the workshop. I wanted them all. I had five in my hands. A friend looked at me and laughed.

"Get more," she said.

"I would, but there will be a reckoning when I return to real life."

A woman nearby overheard. "This is your real life," she said. "All of it."

I thought again of my almost stealing those wings. I was glad I gave them back. When I flew home, I returned with twelve books. I hugged my children. I made no apologies. I was glad for the week. I was glad to be back. I know I do my best work surrounded by the waffles, the bent pages of feminist theory, bright plastic cars, and silver wands.

ACKNOWLEDGMENTS

When I began this book, I was one kind of mother: married, homebound; the kind who did crafts and planned elaborate parties. When I finished this book, I was another kind of mother: divorced, working all the time; when I planned parties, I barely even remembered to buy cake. It changed the way I saw myself as a mother. It changed how I saw my own mother. So many people say you need to have kids to understand your mother. I say you have to get divorced.

What I understood about my mother was how alone she was. What I understood about motherhood is how alone we all are. How, even now, the experience of motherhood is so transforming and isolating, each of us feels as if we've discovered something new every time we do it.

I write all of this to put into context the enormous labor of the people in my life who made me become me and helped me write this book. The women who shared their stories and research, fears, and rages. And the women who will keep sharing and sharing until we can tell a new story. These women are Anna Marsh, Kate Johansen, KT Bukowski, who know and love me no matter what form I take. Kristin Engel, Melanie Ostmo, Yara Conway, Jessie Jones, Katie Hallman, Beth Papendick, every single Witch on Facebook, Maria Guido, Sarah Weinman, Kerry Howley, Rachel Yoder, and Chloe Angyal. The agent who pushed this book into being, Saba Sulaiman. And my sisters, who are all versions of humans I wish I could be.

Special thanks to the men, who know this book is for them, too, and who helped me in so many ways with so many emotional labors. Elon Green and Cavan Hallman. And my brother, who has always told me my story was mine to tell.

To the other men: I wrote this book in spite of you.

Of course, my own mother, who put me in this basket of reeds and sent me down this river. And in whom my cells still mingle. She will always be part of me, and I, her.

Thank you to Jia Tolentino, who let me write about whatever I wanted for *Jezebel* and it turned into this book. Parts of this book are adapted and expanded upon from those early essays. May we all be blessed with editors who say, "Get weirder!"

Remy Cawley spent so much time making this book perfect. She tightened my thoughts and ideas until you could bounce quarters off of them. The love and care she put into this book are the reason it's here. She saw a book where I just saw internet rants. She also made sure this had space for all kinds of mothers.

But, in the end, this book wouldn't be here if I didn't have my children, Ellis and Jude. I want you to know that every time I write something, I'm trying to make the world you live in a little better.

NOTES

Introduction: Who Gets to Be a Mother?

1. Lauren Silverman, "In Texas, Abstinence-Only Programs May Contribute to Teen Pregnancies," NPR, June 5, 2017, www.npr.org/sections/health-shots/2017/06/05/530922642/in-texas-abstinence-only-programs-may-contribute-to-teen-pregnancies.

2. Virginia Sole-Smith, "When You're Told You're Too Fat to Get Pregnant," *New York Times Magazine*, June 18, 2019, www.nytimes.com/2019/06/18/magazine/fertility-weight-obesity-ivf.html.

3. Brianna Snyder, "Fat-Shaming the Pregnant: How the Medical Community Fails Overweight Moms," *Huffington Post*, September 5, 2018, www.huffpost.com/entry/fat-shaming-pregnant-overweight-moms_n_5b89a872e4b0511db3d872a9.

4. Lisa Rapaport, "Half of U.S. Women Are Overweight during Pregnancy," Reuters, July 1, 2015, www.reuters.com/article/us-health-pregnancy-obesity/half-of-u-s-women-are-overweight-during-pregnancy-idUSKCN0PB5DB20150701.

5. Diana Delgado, Interview with Donna Delgado, Women and Prison, accessed January 20, 2020, http://womenandprison.org/interviews/view/interview_with_diana_delgado.

6. *Incarcerated Women and Girls* [fact sheet] (Washington, DC: The Sentencing Project, June 2019), www.sentencingproject.org/wp-content/uploads/2016/02/Incarcerated-Women-and-Girls.pdf.

7. "First of Its Kind Statistics on Pregnant Women in U.S. Prisons," Johns Hopkins Medicine, March 21, 2019, www.hopkinsmedicine.org/news/newsroom/news-releases/first-of-its-kind-statistics-on-pregnant-women-in-us-prisons.

8. Eli Hager and Anna Flagg, "How Incarcerated Parents Are Losing Their Children Forever," The Marshall Project, December 2, 2018, www.themarshallproject.org/2018/12/03/how-incarcerated-parents-are-losing-their-children-forever.

9. Jennifer G. Clarke and Rachel E. Simon, "Shackling and Separation: Motherhood in Prison," *AMA Journal of Ethics* 15, no. 9 (2013): 779–785, https://journalofethics.ama-assn.org/article/shackling-and-separation-motherhood-prison/2013-09.

10. "Incarcerated Women and Girls," The Sentencing Project, June 6, 2019, www.sentencingproject.org/publications/incarcerated-women-and-girls/.

11. "One Mother's Death: Shalon's Story," Health Resources and Services Administration, last reviewed June 2018, www.hrsa.gov/enews/past-issues/2018/july-5/shalons-story.html.

12. Nina Martin and Renee Montagne, "Black Mothers Keep Dying After Giving Birth. Shalon Irving's Story Explains Why," *All Things Considered*, NPR, December 7, 2017, www.npr.org/2017/12/07/568948782/black-mothers-keep-dying-after-giving-birth-shalon-irvings-story-explains-why.

13. Amy Roeder, "America Is Failing Its Black Mothers," *Harvard Public Health*, Winter 2019, www.hsph.harvard.edu/magazine/magazine_article/america-is-failing-its-black-mothers/.

14. Cristina Novoa and Jamila Taylor, "Exploring African Americans' High Maternal and Infant Death Rates," Center for American Progress, February 1, 2018, www.americanprogress.org/issues/early-childhood/reports/2018/02/01/445576/exploring-african-americans-high-maternal-infant-death-rates/.

15. Roeder, "America Is Failing Its Black Mothers," www.hsph.harvard.edu/magazine/magazine_article/america-is-failing-its-black-mothers/.

16. Stephanie Buckhanon Crowder, *When Momma Speaks: The Bible and Motherhood from a Womanist Perspective* (Louisville, KY: Westminster John Knox Press, 2016), 8.

17. Lisa Wade, "Sterilization of Women of Color: Does 'Unforced' Mean 'Freely Chosen'?" *Ms.*, July 21, 2011, https://msmagazine.com/2011/07/21/sterilization-of-women-of-color-does-unforced-mean-freely-chosen/.

18. Trevor Burrus, "The Crackpot Craze That Sterilized 60,000 American Women and Men," *Newsweek*, January 30, 2016, www.newsweek.com/crackpot-craze-sterilized-60000-american-women-men-421300.

19. Saudi Garcia, "8 Shocking Facts About Sterilization in U.S. History," *Mic*, July 10, 2013, www.mic.com/articles/53723/8-shocking-facts-about-sterilization-in-u-s-history#.2HykXjWH2.

20. Lea Hunter, "The U.S. Is Still Forcibly Sterilizing Prisoners," Talk Poverty, August 23, 2017, https://talkpoverty.org/2017/08/23/u-s-still -forcibly-sterilizing-prisoners/.

21. Miranda Bryant, "Alabama: Pregnant Woman Shot in Stomach Is Charged in Fetus's Death," *The Guardian*, June 27, 2019, www.theguardian .com/us-news/2019/jun/27/alabama-pregnant-woman-shot-manslaughter -charge-marshae-jones.

22. Isha Aran, "Woman Who Left Kids in Car During Job Interview Regains Custody," Jezebel, September 2, 2014, https://jezebel.com/woman -who-left-kids-in-car-during-job-interview-regains-1629662235.

23. Diamond Sharp, "Black Mothers Under Siege," The Root, August 5, 2014, www.theroot.com/black-mothers-under-siege-1790868446.

24. Lara Americo, "I'm a Trans Woman Who Detransitioned to Become a Mom," Them, May 13, 2018, www.them.us/story/im-a-trans-woman-who -detransitioned-to-become-a-mom.

25. Lara Americo, "Four Puberties, One Baby," Parenting, *New York Times*, June 11, 2019, https://parenting.nytimes.com/becoming-a-parent /transgender-fertility-pregnant.

26. Isabel Gregg, "The Health Care Experiences of Lesbian Women Becoming Mothers," *Nursing for Women's Health*, 22, no. 1 (2018), 40–50, https:// nwhjournal.org/article/S1751-4851(17)30333-1/fulltext#s0050.

27. "Same-Sex Parenting in the U.S." [press release], The Williams Institute, UCLA, July 31, 2018, https://williamsinstitute.law.ucla.edu/press /press-releases/same-sex-parenting/.

28. Mary Wollstonecraft, *A Vindication of the Rights of Woman* (London: J. Johnson, 1796), https://archive.org/details/avindicationrig01wollgoog/page /n3/mode/2up.

Conception

1. Art Swift, "In U.S., Belief in Creationist View of Humans at New Low," Gallup, May 22, 2017, https://news.gallup.com/poll/210956/belief -creationist-view-humans-new-low.aspx.

2. Barbara C. Sproul, *Primal Myths: Creation Myths from Around the World* (New York: Harper One, 1991), 238.

3. Sproul, *Primal Myths*, 92.

4. Sproul, *Primal Myths*, 188.

5. Rebecca Kukla, *Mass Hysteria: Medicine, Culture, and Mothers' Bodies* (Lanham, MD: Rowman & Littlefield, 2005), 108.

6. Georgi Boorman, "Is Abortion Really Necessary for Treating Ectopic Pregnancies?" *The Federalist*, September 9, 2019, https://

thefederalist.com/2019/09/09/is-abortion-really-necessary-for-treating-ectopic
-pregnancies/.

7. Harry A. Blackmun, "Supreme Court's Response to the Question: When Does Life Begin? *Roe v. Wade* 1973, Opinion of the Court written by Supreme Court Justice Blackmun," United States Conference of Catholic Bishops, www.usccb.org/issues-and-action/human-life-and-dignity/abortion /supreme-courts-response-to-the-question-when-does-life-begin.cfm.

8. Laura Bassett, "Paul Ryan Cosponsors New Fetal Personhood Bill," Politics, *Huffington Post*, January 9, 2013, www.huffingtonpost.com/2013/01 /09/paul-ryan-personhood-bill_n_2440365.html.

Virgin

1. Christine Emba, "The Dramatic Implosion of 'I Kissed Dating Goodbye' Is a Lesson—and a Warning," Opinions, *Washington Post*, November 14, 2018, www.washingtonpost.com/opinions/the-dramatic-implosion-of-i -kissed-dating-goodbye-is-a-lesson--and-a-warning/2018/11/14/eeecd65c -e850-11e8-bbdb-72fdbf9d4fed_story.html.

2. Thomas Schreiner, "Mary, Did You Know? What the Catholic Church Teaches About the Mother of Jesus," Desiring God, December 23, 2017 www .desiringgod.org/articles/mary-did-you-know.

3. Roger Ebert, "Demi Moore Interview," Roger Ebert Interviews, October 21, 1991 www.rogerebert.com/interviews/demi-moore-interview.

4. Jessica Valenti, *The Purity Myth: How America's Obsession with Virginity Is Hurting Young Women* (Berkeley, CA: Seal Press, 2010), 21.

5. Ambroise Paré, *On Monsters and Marvels*, trans. Janis L. Pallister (Chicago: University of Chicago Press, 1982), 33.

6. Carol Roye, "What Exactly Is a Hymen?" Our Bodies Our Selves, December 14, 2008, last revised March 21, 2014, www.ourbodiesourselves.org /book-excerpts/health-article/what-exactly-is-a-hymen/.

7. Merlin Stone, *When God Was a Woman* (New York: Barnes and Noble Books, 1976), 11.

8. Mathilde Vaerting and Mathias Vaerting, *The Dominant Sex* (New York: George H. Doran, 1923), 160.

9. Stone, *When God Was a Woman*, 20.

10. Stone, *When God Was a Woman*, 21.

11. Hanne Blank, *Virgin: The Untouched History* (New York: Bloomsbury, 2007), 35.

12. Pam Belluck, "Trump Administration Pushes Abstinence in Teen Pregnancy Programs," *New York Times*, April 23, 2018, www.nytimes.com /2018/04/23/health/trump-teen-pregnancy-abstinence.html.

13. "Abstinence Education Programs: Definition, Funding, and Impact on Teen Sexual Behavior," Kaiser Family Foundation, June 1, 2018, www .kff.org/womens-health-policy/fact-sheet/abstinence-education-programs -definition-funding-and-impact-on-teen-sexual-behavior.

14. Joel R. Anderson, Elise Holland, Courtney Heldreth, and Scott P. Johnson, "Revisiting the Jezebel Stereotype: The Impact of Target Race on Sexual Objectification," *Psychology of Women Quarterly* 42 (2018): 461–476, https://doi.org/10.1177/0361684318791543.

15. Mariarosa Dalla Costa and Selma James, *The Power of Women and the Subversion of Community* (Bristol, England: Falling Wall Press, 1971).

16. Amy H. Herring, Samantha M. Attard, Penny Gordon-Larsen, William H. Joyner, and Carolyn T. Halpern, "Like a Virgin (Mother): Analysis of Data from a Longitudinal, US Population Representative Sample Survey," *BMJ* 347 (2013): f7102, www.bmj.com/content/347/bmj.f7102.

17. "Statistics—Stop Street Harassment Studies," Stop Street Harassment, accessed January 20, 2020, www.stopstreetharassment.org/resources /statistics/sshstudies/.

18. Isak Dinesen, "The Blank Page," *Last Tales* (New York: Random House, 1957; New York: Vintage Books, 1991).

Miscarriage

1. Marina Krakovsky, "Private Loss Visible," *Monitor on Psychology* 37, no. 8 (September 2006): 50, www.apa.org/monitor/sep06/loss.

2. Associated Press, "Woman Accused of Feticide Is Released from Prison," *Indy Star*, September 1, 2016, updated September 2, 2016, www .indystar.com/story/news/crime/2016/09/01/purvi-patel-releases-feticide -conviction-overturned/89707582/.

3. Michael Le Page, "Women Have More Miscarriages Than Live Births Over Their Lifetime," *New Scientist*, July 30, 2018, www.newscientist.com /article/2175534-women-have-more-miscarriages-than-live-births-over -their-lifetime/.

4. J. Bardos, D. Hercz, J. Friedenthal, S. A. Missmer, and Z. Williams, "A National Survey on Public Perceptions of Miscarriage," *Obstetrics and Gynecology* 125, no. 6 (2015): 1313–1320, www.ncbi.nlm.nih.gov/pubmed/26000502.

5. Elisabeth Badinter, *Mother Love: Myth and Reality* (Paris: Flammarion, 1980), 61.

6. "The Brandeis Brief—in Its Entirety," Louis D. Brandeis School of Law Library, accessed January 20, 2020, https://louisville.edu/law/library /special-collections/the-louis-d.-brandeis-collection/the-brandeis-brief -in-its-entirety.

7. Josiah Morris Slemons, *The Prospective Mother: A Handbook for Women during Pregnancy* (New York: D. Appleton and Company, 1921), 132.

8. Claudia Goldin, "Female Labor Force Participation: The Origin of Black and White Differences, 1870 and 1880," *Journal of Economic History* 37, no. 1 (1977): 87–108, https://dash.harvard.edu/bitstream/handle/1/2643657 /Goldin_FemaleLabor.pdf?sequence=4&isAllowed=y.

9. Dalla Costa and James, *Power of Women*.

10. Dalla Costa and James, *Power of Women*.

11. C. J. Bayer, *Maternal Impressions: A Study in Child Life* (1897; repr. Whitefish, MT: Kessinger Publishing, 2006).

12. J. Van Os and J. Selten, "Prenatal Exposure to Maternal Stress and Subsequent Schizophrenia: The May 1940 Invasion of the Netherlands," *British Journal of Psychiatry* 172, no. 4 (1998): 324–326, doi:10.1192/bjp.172.4.324; Nancy Dole, D. A. Savitz, Irve Hertz-Picciotto, A. M. Siega-Riz, M. J. Mc-Mahon, and P. Buekens, "Maternal Stress and Preterm Birth," *American Journal of Epidemiology* 157, no. 1 (January 2003): 14–24, doi:10.1093/aje/kwf176.

13. Michel Martin, "Racism Is Literally Bad for Your Health," *All Things Considered*, NPR, October 28, 2017, www.npr.org/2017/10/28/560444290 /racism-is-literally-bad-for-your-health.

14. "Why Do People Get So Bent Out of Shape About Drinking While Pregnant?" NPR, October 26, 2015, https://www.npr.org/sections/health -shots/2015/10/26/450598553/why-do-people-get-so-bent-out-of-shape -about-drinking-while-pregnant.

15. Lyanne A. Guarecuco, "Lawmaker: Criminalizing Abortion Would Force Women to Be 'More Personally Responsible,'" *Texas Observer*, January 23, 2017, www.texasobserver.org/texas-lawmaker-no-abortion-access-would -force-women-to-be-more-personally-responsible-with-sex/.

Hunger

1. U. Ekwochi, C. D. Osuorah, I. K. Ndu, C. Ifediora, I. N. Asinobi, and C. B. Eke, "Food Taboos and Myths in South Eastern Nigeria: The Belief and Practice of Mothers in the Region," *Journal of Ethnobiology and Ethnomedicine* 12 (2016): 7, www.ncbi.nlm.nih.gov/pubmed/26818243.

2. Nicole Washington, "Eat This, Not That: Taboos and Pregnancy," *National Geographic*, March 15, 2015, www.nationalgeographic.com /people-and-culture/food/the-plate/2015/03/19/eat-this-not-that-taboos -and-pregnancy/.

3. Emily Oster, *Expecting Better: Why the Conventional Pregnancy Wisdom Is Wrong—and What You Really Need to Know* (New York: Penguin, 2014), 53.

4. Omar Manejwala, "What Really Causes Pregnancy Cravings?" *Psychology Today*, June 11, 2013, www.psychologytoday.com/us/blog/craving/201306/what-really-causes-pregnancy-cravings.

5. "Pregnancy and Pica," American Pregnancy Association, accessed January 20, 2020, https://americanpregnancy.org/pregnancy-health/unusual-cravings-pica/.

6. J. F. Pope, J. D. Skinner, and B. R. Carruth, "Cravings and Aversions of Pregnant Adolescents," *Journal of the American Dietetic Association* 92, no. 12 (1992): 1479–1482, www.ncbi.nlm.nih.gov/pubmed/1452960.

7. C. N. Nyaruhucha, "Food Cravings, Aversions and Pica among Pregnant Women in Dar es Salaam, Tanzania," *Tanzania Journal of Health Research* 11, no. 1 (2009): 29–34, www.ncbi.nlm.nih.gov/pubmed/19445102.

8. Yvette Manes, "Pregnancy Cravings Are Real—Here Are Some of the Weirdest Ones, *Insider*, December 8, 2017, www.thisisinsider.com/weirdest-pregnancy-cravings-2017-12#some-wanted-antacids-11.

9. MoshD, "What Is the Reality behind Cross Legs in Pregnancy?" Baby Center, March 13, 2012, www.babycenter.in/thread/41063/what-is-the-reality-behind-cross-legs-in-pregnancy.

10. "Keeping Good Posture During Pregnancy," Ask Dr. Sears, accessed January 20, 2020, www.askdrsears.com/topics/pregnancy-childbirth/pregnancy-concerns/pregnancy-posture.

11. R. Pinar, S. Ataalkin, and R. Watson, "The Effect of Crossing Legs on Blood Pressure in Hypertensive Patients," *Journal of Clinical Nursing* 19, nos. 9–10 (2010): 1284–1288, www.ncbi.nlm.nih.gov/pubmed/20500337; R. Pinar, N. Sabuncu, A. Oksay, "Effects of Crossed Leg on Blood Pressure," Blood Pressure 13, no. 4 (2004): 252–254, www.ncbi.nlm.nih.gov/pubmed/15581341.

12. Valerie Steele, *The Corset: A Cultural History* (New Haven, CT: Yale University Press, 2003), 76.

13. Steele, *The Corset*, 77.

14. Tamara Abraham, "Should Kate Give Up the Stilettos? Duchess of Cambridge's Grate Escape Sparks Debate About Risks of Heels during Pregnancy," *Daily Mail*, March 19, 2013, updated March 20, 2013, www.dailymail.co.uk/femail/article-2296016/Kate-Middleton-pregnant-Should-Duchess-Cambridge-high-heels.html.

15. Hippocrates, *Oevres Complètes d'Hippocrate*, Vol. 8 (Paris: Baillière, 1839), 487.

16. Ambroise Paré, *On Monsters and Marvels*, trans. Janis L. Pallister (Chicago: University of Chicago Press, 1982), 39.

17. Aiden MacFarlane, *The Psychology of Childbirth (The Developing Child)* (Cambridge, MA: Harvard University Press, 1977), 6.

18. Adrienne Rich, *Of Woman Born: Motherhood as Experience and Institution* (New York: W. W. Norton, 1995), 44.

19. Oster, *Expecting Bette*, 146.

20. Jill Hammer, *Sisters at Sinai: New Tales of Biblical Women* (Philadelphia: Jewish Publication Society, 2004), 10.

Desire

1. Caitlin Keating, "Colorado Mother Says She Still 'Yearns' for Baby Girl Aurora Who Died After Being Cut from Her Womb," *People*, February 29, 2016, https://people.com/human-interest/michelle-wilkins-colorado-woman-whose-baby-was-cut-from-her-womb-speaks-out/.

2. Keagan Harsha, "Man Describes Girlfriend's Elaborate Ruse in Dynel Lane's Trial," Fox News, February 17, 2016, updated February 18, 2016, https://kdvr.com/2016/02/17/man-describes-girlfriends-elaborate-ruse-in-dynel-lanes-trial/.

3. Chuck Hickey, "Emotional Michelle Wilkins Describes Attack in First Day of Dynel Lane Trial," Fox News, February 17, 2016, https://kdvr.com/2016/02/17/michelle-wilkins-takes-stand-in-first-day-of-dynel-lane-trial/.

4. Nara Schoenberg, "Women Who Try to Cut Fetuses from Expectant Mothers: Why Do They Do It?" *Chicago Tribune*, February 26, 2016, www.chicagotribune.com/lifestyles/health/sc-women-pregnancy-issues-family-0225-20160225-story.html.

5. Kerry E. Arquette, "Fetal Attraction: A Descriptive Study of Patterns in Fetal Abductions," *All Regis University Theses* 245 (2012), https://epublications.regis.edu/cgi/viewcontent.cgi?article=1245&context=theses.

6. Habek Dubravko, "Pseudocyesis in Peri- and Postmenopausal Women," *Central European Journal of Medicine* 5, no. 3 (2010): 373–374, www.degruyter.com/downloadpdf/j/med.2010.5.issue-3/s11536-009-0084-8/s11536-009-0084-8.pdf.

7. Margaret Sullivan, "Gender Questions Arise in Obituary of Rocket Scientist and Her Beef Stroganoff," Opinion, *New York Times*, April 1, 2013, https://web.archive.org/web/20141208234834/https://publiceditor.blogs.nytimes.com/2013/04/01/gender-questions-arise-in-obituary-of-rocket-scientist-and-her-beef-stroganoff/.

8. Rachel Cusk, "Can a Woman Who Is an Artist Ever Just Be an Artist?" *New York Times Magazine*, November 7, 2019, www.nytimes.com/2019/11/07/magazine/women-art-celia-paul-cecily-brown.html.

9. Judith Butler, *Gender Trouble: Tenth Anniversary Edition* (New York: Routledge, 2002), 14.

10. Esther Fuchs, "The Literary Characterization of Women in the Hebrew Bible," *Feminist Perspectives on Biblical Scholarship*, ed. Adela Yarbro Collins (Chico, CA: Scholars Press, 1985), 117–136.

11. Sigrid Nunez, "The Most Important Thing," in *Selfish, Shallow, and Self-Absorbed: Sixteen Writers on the Decision Not to Have Kids*, ed. Meghan Daum (New York: Macmillan, 2015), 110.

12. Margaret Atwood, *The Handmaid's Tale* (New York: Houghton Mifflin Harcourt, 1986), 24.

Sanity

1. Craig H. Kinsley, Lisa Madonia, Gordon W. Gifford, Kara Tureski, Garrett R. Griffin, Catherine Lowry, Jamison Williams, Jennifer Collins, Heather McLearie, and Kelly G. Lambert, "Motherhood Improves Learning and Memory," *Nature* 402 (1999): 137–138, www.nature.com/articles/45957.

2. Craig H. Kinsley and Kelly G. Lambert, "The Maternal Brain," *Scientific American*, January 2006, www.scientificamerican.com/article/the -maternal-brain/#.

3. Emily Brontë, *Wuthering Heights* (1847; repr. New York: Penguin Books, 2003).

4. Brontë, *Wuthering Heights*.

5. Clare Hanson, *A Cultural History of Pregnancy* (New York: Springer, 2004), 115.

6. David Jacobson, "Study Finds Depression in Pregnancy, Postpartum Is Overlooked and Undertreated," School of Pharmacy, University of California San Francisco, December 1, 2014, https://pharmacy.ucsf.edu/news/2014/12 /study-finds-depression-pregnancy-postpartum-overlooked-undertreated.

7. Sara L. Johansen, Thalia K. Robakis, Katherine Ellie Williams, and Natalie L. Rasgon, "Management of Perinatal Depression with Non-drug Interventions," *BMJ* 364 (2019): 1322, www.bmj.com/content/364/bmj.l322.

8. John B. Tuke, "Cases Illustrative of the Insanity of Pregnancy, Puerperal Mania, and Insanity of Lactation," *Edinburgh Medical Journal* 12, no. 12 (June 1867): 1083–1101, www.ncbi.nlm.nih.gov/pmc/articles/PMC5308353 /pdf/edinbmedj73885-0023.pdf.

9. John Abbott, *The Mother at Home* (Worcester, MA: Crocker & Brewster, 1833; CreateSpace Independent Publisher, 2012).

10. "The Wandering Womb: Female Hysteria through the Ages," Dr. Lindsey Fitzharris, www.drlindseyfitzharris.com/2017/04/28/the-wandering -womb-female-hysteria-through-the-ages/#f1.

11. Rebecca Kukla, *Mass Hysteria: Medicine, Culture, and Mothers' Bodies* (Lanham, MD: Rowman & Littlefield, 2005), 67.

Depths

1. "The Curious Case of Mary Toft, 1726," University of Glasgow Library Special Collections Department, August 2009, http://special.lib.gla.ac.uk/exhibns/month/aug2009.html.

2. Randi Hutter Epstein, *Get Me Out: A History of Childbirth from the Garden of Eden to the Sperm Bank* (New York: W. W. Norton, 2011), 26.

3. Thomas P. Duffy, "The Flexner Report—100 Years Later," *Yale Journal of Biology and Medicine* 84, no. 3 (2011): 269–276, www.ncbi.nlm.nih.gov/pmc/articles/PMC3178858/; "1798: Marine Hospital Service," MCH Timeline, https://mchb.hrsa.gov/about/timeline/timeline-scrn-rdrs.html.

4. Rich, *Of Woman Born*.

5. Alan F. Dixson and Barnaby J. Dixson, "Venus Figurines of the European Paleolithic: Symbols of Fertility or Attractiveness?" *Journal of Anthropology* 2011 (2011): article ID 569120, www.hindawi.com/journals/janthro/2011/569120/.

6. "It's Vitally Important to #KnowYourBody," The Eve Appeal, https://eveappeal.org.uk/news-awareness/know-your-body/.

7. Emma L. E. Rees, *The Vagina: A Literary and Cultural History* (New York: Bloomsbury Academic, 2015).

8. Jan Bondeson, *A Cabinet of Medical Curiosities* (New York: W. W. Norton, 1999).

9. Nina Martin and Renee Montagne, "The Last Person You'd Expect to Die in Childbirth," ProPublica, March 9, 2019, www.propublica.org/article/die-in-childbirth-maternal-death-rate-health-care-system.

10. Roni Caryn Rabin, "Huge Racial Disparities Found in Deaths Linked to Pregnancy," *New York Times*, May 7, 2019, www.nytimes.com/2019/05/07/health/pregnancy-deaths-.html.

11. Tressie McMillan Cottom, *Thick: And Other Essays* (New York: The New Press, 2018), 87.

12. Joseph Campbell, *The Hero with a Thousand Faces* (Princeton, NJ: Princeton University Press, 1949).

Power

1. Barbara Ehrenreich and Deirdre English, *Witches, Midwives, and Nurses: A History of Women Healers*, 2nd ed. (New York: The Feminist Press at CUNY, 2010).

2. Ehrenreich and English, *Witches, Midwives, and Nurses*.

3. Jules Michelet, *Satanism and Witchcraft* (London: 1863; New York: Kensington Publishing Corp., 1998).

4. Arlie Russell Hochschild, *Strangers in Their Own Land: Anger and Mourning on the American Right* (New York: The New Press, 2016).

5. Keisha La'Nesha Goode, "Birthing, Blackness, and the Body: Black Midwives and Experiential Continuities of Institutional Racism" (PhD diss., CUNY Academic Works, 2014), https://academicworks.cuny.edu/cgi /viewcontent.cgi?article=1422&context=gc_etds.

6. Alicia D. Bonaparte, "The Persecution and Prosecution of Granny Midwives in South Carolina, 1900–1940" (PhD diss., Vanderbilt University, August 2007), https://etd.library.vanderbilt.edu/available/etd-07252007 -122217/unrestricted/bonapartedissertation2007final.pdf.

7. Alice Walker, *The Temple of My Familiar* (1989; repr. New York: Mariner Books, 2010).

8. J. Czarnocka and P. Slade, "Prevalence and Predictors of Post-traumatic Stress Symptoms Following Childbirth," *British Journal of Clinical Psychology* 39, no. 1 (2000): 35–51, www.ncbi.nlm.nih.gov/pubmed/10789027.

9. Rich, *Of Woman Born.*

Pain

1. V. N. Gamble, "Under the Shadow of Tuskegee: African Americans and Health Care," *American Journal of Public Health* 87, no. 11 (1997): 1773–1778, www.ncbi.nlm.nih.gov/pmc/articles/PMC1381160/?page=2.

2. Kelly M. Hoffman, Sophie Trawalter, Jordan R. Axt, and M. Norman Oliver, "Racial Bias in Pain Assessment and Treatment Recommendations, and False Beliefs About Biological Differences between Blacks and Whites," *Proceedings of the National Academy of Sciences of the United States of America* 113, no. 16 (2016): 4296–4301, www.ncbi.nlm.nih.gov/pmc/articles /PMC4843483/.

3. Martin Luther, "The Estate of Marriage," in *Luther's Works*, Vol. 45 (1522; repr. Minneapolis, MN: Fortress Press, 1970).

4. Sharon Howard, "Imagining the Pain and Peril of Seventeenth Century Childbirth: Travail and Deliverance in the Making of an Early Modern World," *Social History of Medicine* 16, no. 3 (2003).

5. S. Lurie, "Euphemia Maclean, Agnes Sampson and Pain Relief during Labour in 16th Century Edinburgh," *Anaesthesia* 59, no. 8 (2004), https://onlinelibrary.wiley.com/doi/full/10.1111/j.1365-2044.2004.03 891.x.

6. Nora Doyle, "Bodies at Odds: The Maternal Body as Lived Experience and Cultural Expression in America, 1750–1850" (PhD diss., University of

North Carolina at Chapel Hill, 2013), https://pdfs.semanticscholar.org/c2c0 /37be453160434c055bdeb36372988f2802a9.pdf.

7. Judith Walzer Leavitt, "Joseph B. DeLee and the Practice of Preventive Obstetrics," American Journal of Public Health 78, no. 10 (1988): 1353–1361, www.ncbi.nlm.nih.gov/pmc/articles/PMC1349440/.

8. Bee Rowlatt, "The Original Suffragette: The Extraordinary Mary Wollstonecraft," *The Guardian*, October 5, 2015, www.theguardian .com/lifeandstyle/womens-blog/2015/oct/05/original-suffragette-mary -wollstonecraft.

9. Rich, *Of Woman Born*.

10. Robab Latifnejad Roudsari, Maryam Zakerihamidi, and Effat Merghati Khoei, "Socio-Cultural Beliefs, Values and Traditions Regarding Women's Preferred Mode of Birth in the North of Iran," *International Journal of Community Based Nursing and Midwifery* 3, no. 3 (2015): 165–176, www.ncbi .nlm.nih.gov/pmc/articles/PMC4495324/.

11. Maria Guido, "Labor Pains: 'The Business of Being Born' Gave Me a Birthing Complex," Mommyish, October 18, 2012, www.mommyish.com /the-business-of-being-born-birth-265/.

12. Wendy Christiaens, Mieke Verhaeghe, and Piet Bracke, "Pain Acceptance and Personal Control in Pain Relief in Two Maternity Care Models: A Cross-National Comparison of Belgium and the Netherlands," *BMC Health Services Research* 10 (2010): 268, www.ncbi.nlm.nih.gov/pmc/articles /PMC2944275/.

Miracles

1. Pamela K. Stone, "Biocultural Perspectives on Maternal Mortality and Obstetrical Death from the Past to the Present," *American Journal of Physical Anthropology* 159, no. S61 (2016), https://onlinelibrary.wiley.com/doi /full/10.1002/ajpa.22906.

2. Virginia Villa, "5 Facts About Vaccines in the U.S.," Pew Research Center, March 19, 2019, www.pewresearch.org/fact-tank/2019/03/19/5-facts -about-vaccines-in-the-u-s/.

3. Carmen Winant, *My Birth* exhibition, image text, Museum of Modern Art, New York, 2018.

4. Winant, *My Birth*.

5. Robyn, "Polly Block, Mormon Midwife Part 1," The Gift of Giving Life, March 25, 2013, http://thegiftofgivinglife.com/polly-block-mormon -midwife-part-1/.

6. Polly Block, *Polly's Birth Book: A Guide to Obstetrics*, 2nd ed. (American Fork, UT: Hearthspun Publishers, 1984).

7. Amazon reviews for *Educated: A Memoir*, by Tara Westover, accessed January 20, 2020, www.amazon.com/Educated-Memoir-Tara-Westover /product-reviews/0399590501/ref=cm_cr_dp_d_show_all_btm?ie=UTF8 &reviewerType=all_reviews.

8. Margaret Atwood, *Dancing Girls* (1977; repr. London: Vintage, 1996).

Ice Diapers

1. Amber Bellazaire and Erik Skinner, "Preventing Infant and Maternal Mortality: State Policy Options," National Conference of State Legislatures, July 3, 2019, www.ncsl.org/research/health/preventing-infant-and -maternal-mortality-state-policy-options.aspx.

2. Sharon Lerner, "Is 40 Weeks the Ideal Maternity Leave Length?" *Slate*, December 22, 2011, https://slate.com/human-interest/2011/12 /maternity-leave-how-much-time-off-is-healthiest-for-babies-and-mothers .html.

3. Jamila Taylor, Cristina Novoa, Katie Hamm, and Shilpa Phadke, "Eliminating Racial Disparities in Maternal and Infant Mortality," Center for American Progress, May 2, 2019, www.americanprogress.org/issues/women /reports/2019/05/02/469186/eliminating-racial-disparities-maternal-infant -mortality/.

4. Melissa Etehad and Jeremy C. F. Lin, "The World Is Getting Better at Paid Maternity Leave. The U.S. Is Not," *Washington Post*, August 13, 2016, www.washingtonpost.com/news/worldviews/wp/2016/08/13 /the-world-is-getting-better-at-paid-maternity-leave-the-u-s-is-not/.

5. "Senator Gillibrand Announces Legislation to Provide Every American Worker with Paid Leave," US Senator Kirsten Gillibrand site, March 18, 2015, www.gillibrand.senate.gov/news/press/release/senator-gillibrand -announces-legislation-to-provide-every-american-worker-with-paid-leave.

6. Christopher J. Ruhm, "Parental Leave and Child Health," *Journal of Health Economics* 19, no. 6 (November 2000): 931–960, http://libres.uncg.edu /ir/uncg/f/C_Ruhm_Parental_2000.pdf.

7. Lerner, "Is 40 Weeks the Ideal Maternity Leave Length?"

8. WHO Department of Maternal, Newborn, Child and Adolescent Health and WHO Department of Reproductive Health and Research, *Postnatal Care for Mothers and Newborns: Highlights from the World Health Organization 2013 Guidelines* (Geneva, Switzerland: World Health Organization, April 2015), www.who.int/maternal_child_adolescent/publications /WHO-MCA-PNC-2014-Briefer_A4.pdf.

9. Presidential Task Force on Redefining the Postpartum Visit, Committee on Obstetric Practice, "Optimizing

Postpartum Care," ACOG Committee Opinion no. 736, May 2018, www
.acog.org/clinical/clinical-guidance/committee-opinion/articles/2018/05
/optimizing-postpartum-care.

10. Jessica Sager, "The Wing's CEO Audrey Gelman Is the First Woman
to Pose Visibly Pregnant on a Business Magazine and It's Amazing AF,"
Parade, September 19, 2019, https://parade.com/925293/jessicasager/the
-wings-ceo-audrey-gelman-is-the-first-woman-to-pose-visibly-pregnant-on
-a-business-magazine-and-its-amazing-af/.

11. Jenn Gann, "The Most 'Real' Scene in Tully Isn't About Horrific
Motherhood," The Cut, *New York Magazine*, May 8, 2018, www.thecut.com
/2018/05/the-most-real-scene-in-tully-charlize-theron-movie-review.html.

12. Brigid Schutte, "The Second Shift at 25: Q & A with Arlie Hochschild," *Washington Post*, August 6, 2014, www.washingtonpost
.com/blogs/she-the-people/wp/2014/08/06/the-second-shift-at-25-q-a
-with-arlie-hochschild/.

Mom Bod

1. Courtney Jung, "We Need to Stop Exaggerating the Benefits of Breastfeeding," The Blog, *Huffington Post*, December 2, 2015, www.huffingtonpost
.ca/courtney-jung/benefits-of-breastfeeding_b_8700120.html.

2. Jacqueline H. Wolf, *Don't Kill Your Baby: Public Health and the Decline
of Breastfeeding in the Nineteenth and Twentieth Centuries* (Columbus: Ohio
State University Press, 2001), 197.

3. Betsy Sussler, ed., "Mary Gaitskill and Matthew Sharpe," Bomb: The
Author Interviews (New York: Soho Press, 2014).

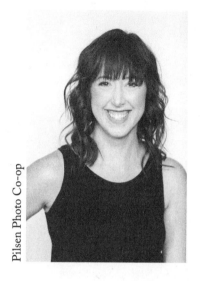

Lyz Lenz is the author of *God Land,* a columnist for the *Cedar Rapids Gazette,* and a contributing writer for the *Columbia Journalism Review.* Her work has also appeared in the *New York Times,* the *Washington Post, Huffington Post,* and *Pacific Standard,* among other publications. She lives in Iowa.